PREVENTION'S

Medical Care
Yearbook
1990

PREVENTION'S

Medical Care Yearbook

1990

Edited by Mark Bricklin, Editor
and Sharon Stocker Ferguson,
Associate Editor
Prevention Magazine

Written by the Staff of Rodale Press

Rodale Press, Emmaus, Pennsylvania

Chapter 5, "The Total Cholesterol Story," was adapted from *Good Fat, Bad Fat*, by Glen C. Griffin, M.D., and William P. Castelli, M.D. (Tucson, Ariz.: Fisher Books, 1989). Reprinted by permission of the publisher.

Chapter 7, "A How-to-Take-Common-Drugs Guide," was adapted from *50+: The Graedons' People's Pharmacy for Older Adults*, by Joe and Theresa Graedon (New York: Bantam Books, 1988). Copyright © 1988 by Graedon Enterprises, Inc. Reprinted by permission of Bantam Books, a division of Bantam Doubleday Dell Publishing Group, Inc. All rights reserved.

The following chapters were adapted from and reprinted by permission of *Medical Self-Care* magazine, P.O. Box 1000, Pt. Reyes, CA 94956 (free sample magazine available on request): chapter 12, "Free Yourself from UTIs" ("No More UTI Misery," January–February 1989); chapter 13, "Make Sure Your 'Pressure' Medicine's Not Squeezing Your Heart" ("Drugs That Hurt the Heart," November–December 1988); chapter 17, "Update on Skin Cancer" ("Fastest Rising Cancer under the Sun," May–June 1988); chapter 23, "Bathe Away Your Winter Blues" ("Don't Be SAD," January–February 1989); chapter 24, "Take Control of Epilepsy" ("Self-Help for Seizures," May–June 1988); and chapter 35, "Uterine Fibroids: Clear Up Your Confusion" ("Uterine Fibroids," July–August 1988).

If you have any questions or comments concerning this book, please write:
Rodale Press
Book Reader Service
33 East Minor Street
Emmaus, PA 18098

ISBN 0-87857-871-4   hardcover

Distributed in the book trade by St. Martin's Press

2 4 6 8 10 9 7 5 3 1   hardcover

Notice

This book is intended as a reference volume only, not as a medical manual or guide to self-treatment. If you suspect that you have a medical problem, we urge you to seek competent medical help. Keep in mind that nutritional and health needs vary from person to person, depending on age, sex, health status, and total diet. The information here is intended to help you make informed decisions about your health, not to substitute for any treatment that may have been prescribed by your doctor.

Contributors to the *Medical Care Yearbook*

WRITERS: Charles Agvent, Kim Anderson, Stefan Bechtel, Pam Boyer, Peggy Jo Donahue, Sid Kirchheimer, Steve Lally, William LeGro, Mike McGrath, Gloria McVeigh, Gale Malesky, Joe Mullich, Cathy Perlmutter, Andrew Roblin, Porter Shimer, Melanie Chadwick Stevens, Stephen Williams, Susan Zarrow

PRODUCTION EDITOR: Jane Sherman

DESIGNER: Glen Burris

COVER DESIGNER: Darlene Schneck

COPY EDITOR: Louise Doucette

EXECUTIVE EDITOR, *PREVENTION* MAGAZINE: Emrika Padus

ASSOCIATE RESEARCH CHIEF, *PREVENTION* MAGAZINE: Pam Boyer

OFFICE MANAGER: Roberta Mulliner

OFFICE PERSONNEL: Eve Buchay, Karen Earl-Braymer

Contents

Introduction
Getting a Third Opinion xvii

Part I
Medical Care Frontiers

Flash Reports
Balloons That Plug Ulcers 1
A Garbage Collector for Arterial Plaque 1
Old Gout Drug Aids Cirrhosis Sufferers 2
Pacemakers for Active People 2

Chapter 1
Science's New Plaque Fighters 3
Today there are more ways than ever to reverse the damage
to arteries clogged with cholesterol and fatty deposits.
Here's a look at the latest, including diet, drugs, angio-
plasty, and bypass surgery.

Chapter 2
The Latest Laser Technology 11
Precise, sterile, bloodless: Lasers are revolutionizing medicine. Some of the laser-treated conditions covered here are
glaucoma, cataracts, skin lesions, birthmarks, endometriosis, infertility, brain tumors, and kidney stones.

Chapter 3
Heart Therapies on the Horizon 19
Scientists make a five-year forecast of the hottest new
trends in heart research, predicting breakthroughs in these
areas: proof of how atherosclerosis actually starts at the
cellular level, life-saving recommendations for LDL and
HDL levels, and clear-cut genetic risk detection.

Chapter 4
Big Miracles in Small Packages 23
Researchers are hard at work on microscopic gears with
shafts one-fifth the width of a human hair and teeth the
size of red blood cells, predicting their possible uses to
scrub arteries clean, create artificial organs, and send pro-
grammed medication into your body.

Chapter 5
The Total Cholesterol Story 26
Heart specialists are learning that, to prevent and treat
heart disease, it's not enough to know only the "total
cholesterol" number. Here, get the straight facts about all
the cholesterol numbers you should know about.

Part II
New State-of-the-Art Treatments

Flash Reports
Arthritis Drug Comes to America 32
New Ultrasound Saves Sight 32
Heart Attack Treatments Team Up 33
Expanding Uses for Balloons 34

Chapter 6
Say Good-Bye to Gallstones 34
Get the complete lowdown from this Q & A on gallstones:
how they form, who's at risk for getting them, what to do
about them, and much more.

Chapter 7
A How-to-Take-Common-Drugs Guide   41
Food can delay or prevent the entry of drugs into the
bloodstream. Here's your guide to which foods block
which medications.

Chapter 8
Don't Put Up With Incontinence   47
Incontinence is not a disease but a symptom of urinary
conditions that can often be cured. Here's information and
advice to help you return to a normal life.

Chapter 9
Update on Intermittent Claudication   54
A report on how you can identify this disease, what you
can expect from your doctor once you're diagnosed, and
which steps to take to gain relief.

Chapter 10
Fighting Dry-Eye Syndrome   61
When not properly treated, this seemingly innocuous disorder can cause serious problems, even blindness. Our
update explains the most common causes and treatments
of dry eyes and takes a look at future technologies.

Chapter 11
Put a Stop to Sinusitis   70
A comprehensive review of the causes of sinus infection
and postnasal drip, preventive measures to take to keep
yourself draining freely, and medical treatments that fix
serious problems once and for all.

Chapter 12
Free Yourself From UTIs   75
A dozen-plus tips for treating and preventing painful
urinary tract infections.

Chapter 13
**Make Sure Your "Pressure" Medicine's Not
Squeezing Your Heart**   78
Here's a report on the newly discovered connection
between certain high blood pressure medications and
increased cholesterol levels.

Chapter 14
Open Your Eyes to New Eyewear Advances 80
New technology in eyeglasses features super-lightweight
lenses, antireflection coatings, and UV-filtering lenses.
Specially designed contact lenses are reshaping eyes and
improving vision.

Part III
Update on Cancer

Flash Reports

Detecting Tiny Tumors 89
High-Tech Machine Zaps Cancer 89
Fighting Bladder Cancer 90
Improving on Breast Surgery 90

Chapter 15
Newest Weapons in the War on Cancer 91
Experts from a world-renowned cancer center, Roswell
Park Memorial Institute in Buffalo, New York, highlight
the latest innovations in cancer prevention, detection, and
treatment.

Chapter 16
**A Guide to America's Best Cancer Treatment
Centers** 97
No matter what part of the country you live in, you'll be
able to use this list to find state-of-the-art treatment at a
top clinic that's close to home.

Chapter 17
Update on Skin Cancer 115
Increasing malignant melanoma rates in North America
could be slowed, stopped, or even decreased by practicing
the simple preventive measures and early detection methods presented here.

Chapter 18
Zap Prostate Cancer 121
Tiny radioactive capsules offer new hope to men with early
cases of prostate cancer. The procedure, which uses only
local anesthesia and is done on an outpatient basis in about
45 minutes, looks promising.

Part IV
The Mind, Nerves, and Health

Flash Reports
Beat the Digitalis Blues 124
Subliminal Messages Speed Recovery 124
Aspirin Reverses Stroke Dementia 125

Chapter 19
New Migraine Tamers 126
Six innovative treatments—from cutting out aspirin to sip-
ping feverfew—are relieving pain for many long-term
sufferers.

Chapter 20
All about Alzheimer's 133
Here's the latest info on what's happening in Alzheimer's
research, plus helpful, compassionate recommendations
on how to care for the patient.

Chapter 21
Sure-to-Soothe Agents for Body and Brain 140
A review of ten on-the-spot tranquilizers from nature and
science.

Chapter 22
Getting Out From Under the Threat of Panic Attacks 149
Who gets these dreaded onslaughts of anxiety and fear,
what seems to cause them, and how to overcome them are
the highlights here.

Chapter 23
Bathe Away Your Winter Blues 159
Daily light baths often cure the winter depression called
seasonal affective disorder. Here's an update on the latest
research.

Chapter 24
Take Control of Epilepsy 161
Yoga, relaxation, and biofeedback can all be used to help
the epileptic learn to dissipate seizures before they strike.
In some cases, medication can even be eliminated.

Part V
Medical Tests and Your Health

Flash Reports
Making Chlamydia Detection Easier 175
Lung Cancer Test of the Future 176
Finding Food Allergies 177

Chapter 25
Update on Osteoporosis Screening 178
While the bone density testing business has boomed in the
past few years, many experts, including the National Osteoporosis Foundation, reject mass screening. Here's how
to find out if a test for you is warranted or not.

Chapter 26
Calming Those Pretest Nerves 183
Two factors can make you anxious about medical tests—
the procedure itself and the results. Here's a guide to
coping with both.

Chapter 27
A New Look at B$_{12}$ Deficiency 189
Evidence is showing that standard tests for this vitamin
aren't accurate, suggesting that deficiency may be more
widespread than previously believed.

Part VI
Better Ways to Beat
Everyday Health Problems

Flash Reports
Comparison Shopping for Dental Fillings 196
Safeguard Your Eyes' Health 197
Keeping Cavities Out 198

Chapter 28
Ten Medicine-Chest Musts 198
Weeding your cabinet of nonessentials and stocking it with
these doctor-recommended helpers will prepare you for
many common ills and spills.

Chapter 29
Triumph Over Back Pain 205
At the University of Miami's Comprehensive Pain and
Rehabilitation Center, people with chronic, debilitating
back trouble emerge virtually pain free.

Chapter 30
50 Facts and Tips to Help Tame Allergies 212
Some of the most effective treatments ever known have
been all but forgotten as the management of allergy becomes increasingly complex, says one famous allergist.
Here he reveals the simple truths.

Chapter 31
Snore No More 224
One of these nine bed-tested antisnoring treatments should
help you (and your spouse) enjoy a good night's sleep.

Chapter 32
Best Remedies for Fighting Phlegm 228
From chicken soup to exercise to over-the-counter cough
medicines, you'll find out what really works to break up
chest congestion.

Chapter 33
Help for Heel Pain 232
Plantar fasciitis, a common cause of sore heels, can sneak
up on you slowly. By the time you realize it's there, it's
bad. Luckily, this guide will help you catch it early.

Chapter 34
Antihistamine Advice That Won't Start You Snoring 239
Experts tell how they help their patients find medication
that does the job without causing excessive drowsiness.

Part VII
Men's and Women's Health Newsfront

Flash Reports
Getting the Best Breast Cancer Therapy 244
The Pill: Exercise Caution 245
Blood Pressure Drug Preserves Potency 245
Ultra Prostate Care with Ultrasound 246

Chapter 35
Uterine Fibroids: Clear Up Your Confusion 247
Most fibroids cause no problems and can be left alone. But
those that cause heavy bleeding or grow uncomfortably
large usually need treatment. Here's a rundown of your
best options.

Chapter 36
**What Every Woman Should Know about
Hysterectomy** 249
Some physicians and consumer groups feel that many
hysterectomies are unnecessary. If you find yourself in one
of the situations listed here, you should explore the alternatives before you say yes.

Chapter 37
New Cures for Impotence 260
Bad eating and drinking habits are just one of six possible
contributers to impotence that are revealed here. Once you
shape up your act, you're likely to find yourself virile as
ever.

Chapter 38
Update on Minoxidil, the Hair Saver 265
Now that the baldness drug's been on the market for over
a year, dermatologists have a better idea of the its benefits
and drawbacks. Here's the inside story.

Part VIII
Medical Advances
for a More Beautiful You

Flash Reports
Dental Implant Update 270
Don't Let Your Drugs Burn You 271
Chew Your Teeth Whiter 271

Chapter 39
Are You Right for Liposuction? 272
Find out whether or not you're suited for the procedure
that can instantly eradicate bumps and bulges.

Chapter 40
Reduce Wrinkles with Retin-A 276
Advice from the dermatologist who discovered this miracle
medication, including a list of factors you should consider
before starting treatment.

Chapter 41
Battling Blemishes 279
Get rid of oil plugs and acne-causing bacteria that clog
pores with this special cleansing routine.

Chapter 42
New, Beautiful Looks in Dentistry 283
A review of the latest techniques that can make your teeth
stronger and more attractive, including state-of-the-art fillings, porcelain laminates, resin-bonded bridges, and implants—and their approximate costs.

Index 289

Getting
a Third Opinion

If your doctor told you today that you needed your gall-bladder removed, what would you do before saying yes to surgery? My guess is you'd seek a second professional opinion. And you'd be wise to do so.

But if you stopped there, you'd very likely miss out on the best possible medical care, because what you'd really need is a third expert opinion. That's right. And the third expert is *you*.

Blindly handing over decisions about your health to strangers (even M.D.'s) compromises the best possible outcome. (If that were best, we could just write "see your physician" under each chapter title in this book and be done.) After all, you're the one who lives in your body. You're the one who knows whether you're likely to stick with that low-sodium follow-up diet, or not. You're the one with insider information. And you're the one who needs to make the ultimate decisions.

Sure it's easier to look to the doctor to tell you what's wrong, why it hurts, and what you should do. But it's not best.

What's best is getting the facts in order to fully explore the options. Then "expert number three" can consult with experts one and two to define the best possible treatment.

And that's the goal of the *Medical Care Yearbook* for 1990:
helping you become your own best expert.
  Here's to the best possible outcome.

Sharon Stocker Ferguson
Associate Editor
Prevention Magazine

PART I:
MEDICAL CARE FRONTIERS

Flash Reports

BALLOONS
THAT PLUG ULCERS

A quick, easy technique is being tested to stop bleeding from duodenal ulcers, a potentially life-threatening condition that often requires blood transfusion and emergency surgery. A balloon is fitted over an endoscope (flexible tube) and inserted into the upper portion of the small intestine (duodenum), the site of most bleeding ulcers. When inflated, it applies direct pressure, stopping the bleeding. It is then easily deflated and removed. The balloon is still in the experimental stage in Britain and is not being used in the United States yet, says Stephen Holt, M.D., of Southern Illinois University School of Medicine, who collaborated with British surgeon Dr. T. Vincent Taylor in developing the technique.

A GARBAGE COLLECTOR
FOR ARTERIAL PLAQUE

Scientists have discovered that when phospholipids (natural components of cell membranes) are dispersed into saline (salt) solution, they form little spheres filled with water. When these spheres, called liposomes, are injected into the bloodstream, they pick up cholesterol from the artery walls and take it away for disposal in the liver. Early studies on animals showed a dramatic reduction in arterial

1

plaque. Now studies are being conducted on animals that develop atherosclerosis in almost the same way as humans. If liposomes reduce atherosclerosis in animals, that could pave the way for human studies, says Kevin J. Williams, M.D., assistant professor of medicine at Columbia University in New York City.

OLD GOUT DRUG
AIDS CIRRHOSIS SUFFERERS

A centuries-old drug used to treat victims of gout has now been reported to double the survival rate of people with mild to moderate cirrhosis. The disease, which is gradually debilitating, has no cure so far. Researchers at the National Institute of Nutrition in Mexico City tested the drug, colchicine, against a placebo (inactive pill) in 100 patients. After five years, 75 percent of those treated with colchicine were still alive, compared with only 34 percent of those given the placebo. After ten years, 56 percent of those taking the drug were still alive, versus only 20 percent in the placebo group.

PACEMAKERS
FOR ACTIVE PEOPLE

Traditionally, pacemakers ran at one speed only. They beat at a slow, steady pace that was fine at rest but lagged behind if you tried to exercise. A few years ago, pacemakers that sensed body motion arrived. They were an important improvement. Now there's a new generation of sophisticated pacemakers that really can match your body's needs, at rest or at play.

One device responds to the number of breaths you take per minute. Another actually responds to the behavior of the heart itself, using the electrical signals of the cardiac tissue to determine the need for an increase or decrease in heart rate.

One caution: Before you agree to a pacemaker, make

sure you get a second opinion! A recently published study shows that at least 20 percent of pacemakers aren't needed.

CHAPTER 1

Science's New Plaque Fighters

Top cardiologists reveal the latest artery-clearing techniques, from diet and drugs to balloons and bypasses.

What's soft and gooey on the outside, tough and gritty on the inside, and can have the effect of a seven-car pileup in rush-hour traffic?

Give up?

The answer is plaque, an artery-clogging mass of fat, cholesterol, calcium, blood-clotting substances, and cellular waste. Over time, plaque can build up, narrowing arteries and choking off blood flow. Angina, or chest pain, verifies its presence. In the worst scenario, a heart attack or stroke may ensue. No one knows exactly why plaque accumulates inside artery walls. Experts believe blood fats and other substances begin to collect when an otherwise smooth artery is damaged, possibly due to factors such as smoking or high blood pressure. Like a nick in crystal glass, a snag in an artery collects debris. And of course, the higher the level of cholesterol in your blood, the greater your chances that fatty plaque deposits will cling to damaged artery walls.

Plaque prevention, then, is clear-cut: Quit smoking, watch your blood pressure, and keep your cholesterol in check. If your arteries are already plastered with plaque, however, you may need to take more aggressive actions to clear your lifelines. The good news is that there are more ways than ever to reverse the damage that's already been done. Read on.

Lifestyle Changes

No one knows for certain what constitutes a plaque reversal diet. But at a recent American Heart Association conference, Dean Ornish, M.D., director of the Preventive Medicine Research Institute in Sausalito, California, presented preliminary findings that may help point the way to a plaque-attack diet, or a plaque-attack lifestyle.

One group in the 50-person study followed a plaque-clearing regimen: They ate a strict vegetarian diet with just 8 to 10 percent of total calories from fat, mostly unsaturated; walked an hour a day, three times a week; and practiced meditation techniques for an hour a day. Those who smoked quit. (In case you're wondering, stress reduction is important because cholesterol is a building block for many of the stress hormones. So if you're chronically under stress, your body may keep churning out too much cholesterol.)

The control group was advised (but not required) to make moderate lifestyle changes to lower cholesterol and control blood pressure. That is, they were given the kind of general information most doctors give to their patients with coronary risk factors.

After one year, the 12 people evaluated in the test group had an average total cholesterol drop from 213 to 151. Their average coronary artery blockages decreased from 44.4 percent to 40.8 percent. What's more, Dr. Ornish points out, some individual arteries had far more dramatic changes, since all patients had at least one artery that was narrowed by 70 percent or more.

In the control group, the 17 people so far tested had less significant changes in their cholesterol levels. And average artery blockages increased from 44.1 percent to 46.2 percent. Exactly how a radical cholesterol-lowering lifestyle zaps plaque is admittedly unclear.

"In simple terms, the body has a great capacity to heal

itself if we give it a chance," says Dr. Ornish. "But if three times a day we're putting more fat and cholesterol into the body than it can metabolize, then it never gets a chance to heal itself."

Your total cholesterol level is a rough gauge for which plaque-bashing steps you may need. There's really no magic number. But a high total cholesterol reading (certainly above 200, perhaps much lower) may be a danger sign. In any case, it's a sure bet that the diet you'll need to reverse plaque will be far more stringent than the diet you'd need to prevent it.

In a famous University of Southern California (USC) study comparing the effects of diet alone to those of diet plus cholesterol-lowering drugs, a low-fat diet did reduce plaque buildup in 2.4 percent of the persons tested. And that diet was less restrictive than Dr. Ornish's, taking 26 percent of its total calories from fat.

The vegetarian diet from Dr. Ornish's study has the bare minimum of fat intake to meet your body's needs. If you want to follow the diet, you'll have to cut out all animal products except egg whites and consume a cup a day of nonfat milk or yogurt. Beyond that, you'll need to limit "good" fatty foods like avocados, nuts, seeds, and soybeans. Added oils are forbidden. Otherwise, you can eat all the fruits, vegetables, grains, and legumes you want.

Remember that this diet, while promising, is not yet proven. And some doctors recommend that patients who go on such diets do so under medical supervision, especially since there is debate whether this specific diet provides enough calcium for your body's needs. Dr. Ornish says that this diet causes you to excrete less calcium, so the calcium in the cup a day of nonfat milk or yogurt may be sufficient.

Keep in mind, though, that once you begin, diet and lifestyle changes should be a lifetime process. "It's not something you can do for six months because you're enthusiastic and then slack off," says Linda Cashin-Hemphill, M.D., coauthor of the USC study.

No matter what other steps you take for your plaque— whether bypass surgery or cholesterol-lowering drugs—

be assured that diet will play a part in your treatment. That's because plaque will build up again unless you change the practices that helped to create it in the first place.

Drugs

In recent years, new cholesterol-lowering drugs have come onto the market. As part of a heart disease prevention program, they are considered invaluable—particularly for people with dangerously high blood cholesterol levels that resist dietary control.

And, at least in one study, when diet alone failed to melt away existing plaque, these drugs appeared to do the trick. In the University of Southern California study, 16 percent of the patients who were placed on a low-fat diet (26 percent of calories) and given cholesterol-lowering drugs saw their plaque shrink.

These drugs are not without drawbacks, however. They can cost several thousand dollars a year, and some may produce side effects like nausea and constipation.

"You should be aware, too, that a commitment to cholesterol-lowering drugs is a commitment for life," says Dr. Cashin-Hemphill. "And that surprises some people."

Balloon Angioplasty

The least invasive way to immediately clear a serious blockage is balloon angioplasty. Here, a thin tube (called a catheter) with an inflatable tip is inserted into an artery in your groin or arm. Then doctors, guided by a fluoroscope (intermittent x-ray images projected on a TV monitor), direct the catheter to your plaque blockage. The balloon is briefly inflated, sometimes several times, and the plaque is broken apart and then pressed against the artery wall, opening the channel so that more blood can flow through. The procedure usually takes an hour.

Angioplasty is relatively painless—you'll need only a local anesthetic. In fact, when you're undergoing angioplasty, you can often watch the procedure on the monitor as the catheter snakes its way up to the blockage.

After angioplasty, patients have to stay in the hospital for a couple of days. But they often can go right back to work. The procedure costs about $6,000—roughly one-fifth as much as bypass surgery.

The popularity of angioplasty is ballooning: About 185,000 were performed in the United States in 1987 compared with about 32,000 in 1983. Still, the procedure is not for everyone.

If there is, say, a sharp bend in the artery leading to your blockage, a catheter may be unable to reach it. And if x-rays reveal your plaque contains a lot of hardened calcium, the balloons may be unable to break it open. There's also a 1 to 2 percent mortality rate with angioplasty, depending on the complexity of the situation.

"Angioplasty is replacing bypass surgery in the easier cases," says Thomas L. Robertson, M.D., chief of the Cardiac Diseases Branch, Division of Heart and Vascular Diseases at the National Heart, Lung, and Blood Institute. "But we have a real problem in knowing which procedure is best for patients with multivessel disease involving two or three vessels."

According to new guidelines formulated by the American College of Cardiology and the American Heart Association, you're an "ideal" candidate for angioplasty if you're a man under 65 with an easily accessible blockage in one artery that is noncalcified.

You're considered to be at "greater risk," but still may benefit from angioplasty, if you're a woman over 65 who has already had bypass surgery or has a history of diabetes, high blood pressure, or disease in several arteries.

However, the technology for this procedure is so new that hard-and-fast rules are impossible to formulate. For example, Dr. Robertson believes the evidence is not clear enough to necessarily say you're "at greater risk" if you're a woman.

Angioplasty has another pitfall: restenosis (pronounced RE-ste-NO-sis). This is what occurs when a vessel narrows again. It happens in about three out of every ten angioplasties. However, several promising solutions to restenosis are now being tested. (See "Angioplasty Alert: Future Techniques.")

Angioplasty Alert:
Future Techniques

If you need to undergo angioplasty, ask your doctor about recent technological improvements: Some 40 new angioplasty gadgets, including new types of catheters, are being developed around the country. Here are three promising techniques that may some day solve the ongoing problem of restenosis—when arteries close again.

Fish oil. A recent pilot study with 82 high-risk men showed the benefits of administering fish oil one week before angioplasty. Only 16 percent of arteries in the fish oil group narrowed again within four months, compared with 36 percent of the arteries in a control group. The results must still be confirmed by larger studies. One potential problem is that fish oil can inhibit the blood's ability to clot, and this could cause complications if emergency bypass surgery is needed.

Stents. Imagine inserting a thin tube inside your artery. That tube is called a stent. These meshlike elastic tubes are inserted after angioplasty to keep blood vessels open. The device is still experimental and is now being tested at only a few centers around the United States.

Laser angioplasty. A laser beam inside the catheter can be used to blast away plaque and/or to "weld" or "glaze" the interior artery after the angioplasty. It, too, is being tested at only a few places. "Using lasers to glaze arteries is like painting a coating over the inner wall so the restenosis never has a chance to develop," says Greg Dehmer, M.D., director of the cardiac catheterization lab at the University of North Carolina at Chapel Hill.

Laser-Assisted Angioplasty

If your coronary artery is so clogged with plaque that an uninflated balloon can't squeeze in, you'll have to bypass angioplasty and go right to surgery. That's not necessarily true for blockages in your limbs. In this case, you may be able to benefit from the use of a hot-tip catheter.

This type of catheter has a laser-heated metal tip at its end that burns away enough plaque to make room for the angioplasty balloon. More than 100 centers nationwide now do the procedure. Use of the hot tip for coronary arteries is still experimental, as are other laser procedures for heart disease.

Surgery

There are two main indications that bypass surgery may be necessary: if you have angina (a pain in the chest that feels like a fist clenching your heart) that can't be controlled with drugs like nitroglycerin, or if tests reveal that your heart's ventricle is damaged. As the name *bypass* suggests, this procedure is more of a detour than a cure.

Most bypasses involve the coronary artery, which feeds blood to the heart. In traditional heart bypasses, surgeons remove a vein from your leg (where its work is taken over by other veins). One end of the vein is hooked onto the aorta, your heart's main pump. The other end is attached to the coronary artery at a point past the blockage.

It may sound simple, but don't be fooled. Coronary bypass surgery is a big deal. You must stay in the hospital for six to eight days after surgery, and your recovery period can be two to three months.

It also has about a 2 percent mortality rate, roughly the same as angioplasty, for a single-vessel bypass. Still, that's not bad considering the alternative—a possible stroke, heart attack, or worse.

More good news is that many surgeons are using a new bypass procedure that extends the benefits of the operation. That is, they are using grafts from the chest arteries in addition to, or instead of, grafts from the leg.

For reasons that aren't entirely clear, grafts from chest arteries are less likely to clog than those from leg veins.

"We have seen several patients who have completely open internal thoracic [chest] grafts that were put in 17 years ago," says Floyd D. Loop, M.D., one of the nation's leading thoracic surgeons. "You can't find that kind of longevity with leg grafts."

And because chest-artery grafts offer this advantage over other grafts, you'll have fewer hospitalizations for cardiac causes, a lower rate of subsequent heart attacks, and fewer repeat operations. Still, like any treatment for coronary disease, thoracic grafts have their drawbacks. They often can't be used for emergency operations (because they take more time), and they aren't as versatile as leg-vein grafts. Another promising technique under study is using grafts from the stomach.

"When we operate on coronary disease—whether we use lasers or balloons or bypasses, we're still just temporizing it," says John Eugene, M.D., a cardiovascular surgeon and laser expert at the University of California, Irvine. "The real cause is there and can still come back." What this means, of course, is that even after you undergo bypass or angioplasty, you have to amend your plaque-accumulating ways, whether through exercise or changing your diet. Bypasses, angioplasties, and the like are not cures for heart disease. Rather, they are merely treatments of the symptoms, albeit sometimes lifesaving treatments.

Still, by any measure, the prognosis for people with large amounts of plaque has never been better.

CHAPTER 2

The Latest Laser Technology

Learn how surgeons use concentrated light to vaporize tumors, kidney stones, and more.

A barely tangible beam of light zaps artery-clogging cholesterol, then welds the artery shut. A quick flash restores sight to a man who was virtually blind even after conventional cataract removal surgery. Another beam "energizes" a drug in the body, making cancer cells self-destruct and leaving normal cells unharmed. Scenes from the future? No, just business as usual. These medical procedures are just a few that feature the "star wars" technology of lasers. Some can be performed only at high-tech centers like the Beckman Laser Institute at the University of California, Irvine. Others can be done in your doctor's office. In either case, if lasers are the future, then the future is now.

Anatomy of Laser Power

Just for the record, lasers aren't named after a Dr. Igor Laser or a planet Laser. The word *laser* stands for *light amplification by stimulated emission of radiation*—which means that laser beams are created by stimulating atoms in a "core material" (such as argon gas) to emit "packets" of light, then amplifying and focusing the light in a single beam. Lasers differ from light emitted from an ordinary light bulb because of this greater concentration and intensity and because they consist of a single wavelength, or color, of light. Ordinary light is a mixture of all the colors of the light spectrum and therefore looks white.

Four types of lasers are used regularly in medicine. The argon laser emits a blue or green beam of light and is readily absorbed by red objects—perfect for working on

11

arteries and other tissue containing red hemoglobin. The carbon dioxide (CO_2) laser emits an infrared beam, which vaporizes water. Since our bodies are mostly water, this laser is an efficient cutting tool. The neodymium-YAG (for yttrium, aluminum, and garnet) laser also emits an infrared beam, but at a lower wavelength than the CO_2. The new tunable-dye lasers can be adjusted to the precise wavelength (color) that's best absorbed by whatever is being worked on.

Lasers are impressive in the operating room. They can cut much more precisely than any scalpel. There's less chance of infection because in most cases nothing enters the operating field except a beam of light. A laser cauterizes (seals blood vessels) as it cuts, so less blood is lost. There's less damage to surrounding tissue, so most operation wounds heal better and more quickly. And when used carefully, lasers leave little or no scarring.

In many cases, lasers can be cost-effective, too. Many laser procedures can be done on an outpatient basis, which means no expensive hospital stay and fewer days absent from work.

Lasers do have their limits, though. Laser tonsillectomies, for example, can take 20 minutes—but a good surgeon can use a scalpel to cut them out in 4 or 5 minutes. "In some cases," says one expert, "lasers are just not a good choice."

Sight-Saving Light

Today, lasers are used more by ophthalmologists than by any other specialists. The most common laser procedure is done for diabetic retinopathy, a condition in which tiny extra blood vessels grow in the retina (the back wall of the eye's interior) and into the fluid center of the eye. If not treated in time, these fragile blood vessels rupture and bleed, gradually causing loss of sight. But this slow deterioration can sometimes be stopped by a laser procedure called pan-retinal photocoagulation. The argon laser is used to make anywhere from 3,000 to 6,000 microscopic burns in the retina (destroying about 6 to 10 percent of its total area). This halts the growth of new vessels—and the patient usually notices no additional loss of sight due to the treatment.

Linda Rogers is diabetic. When her ophthalmologist told her she needed laser treatment for retinopathy, she was frightened. But one session changed her mind. "I was surprised at how easy it was," she says. The procedure is usually done over a few sessions—one eye at a time— working from the outer portion in toward the center of the retina. Linda says that her treatments weren't painful, just a bit uncomfortable. "Afterward," she says, "it was like looking through a gray doughnut, but that went away after a few days."

Lasers can also treat another common sight stealer: glaucoma. Fluid inside the eye builds up and causes abnormal pressure. In a procedure called an iridotomy, a laser (usually a YAG) makes a tiny hole in the iris (the eye's colored portion) to drain the fluid. This draining used to be done surgically. But now with lasers it's a painless outpatient procedure that can be done in a matter of minutes—without anesthesia. The same goes for laser trabeculoplasty, a similar procedure on the side of the iris.

One popular misconception is that lasers are used to zap cataracts. They aren't—but they are used *after* a cataract is removed, because the capsule that encloses the lens clouds over in about half of all cases. The YAG laser is used to create a shock wave, which makes a tiny hole in the center of the cloudy capsule through which the eye focuses. Literally, the patient is blind one minute and can see the next. It's a very safe procedure that can save hundreds of dollars per patient because surgery is avoided.

Getting under the Skin

In dermatology and plastic surgery, lasers are used to remove birthmarks, warts, and some precancerous lesions. The oldest procedure in this area is the treatment of port-wine-stain birthmarks, which are caused by an excessive growth of tiny blood vessels just under the skin. According to Bruce M. Achauer, M.D., the chief of plastic surgery at Beckman Laser Institute, the argon laser has been the main treatment for port-wine stains since the early 1970s. The beam passes through the skin and selectively "cooks" the stain so the body can absorb it, fading the mark with little scarring.

But like any other medical procedure, this use of an argon laser has its drawbacks. A local anesthetic must be used, necessitating uncomfortable injections. And the procedure isn't usually used on children because it may produce noticeable scars on their more delicate skin.

Carol Moeller had a port-wine-stain birthmark for 40 years before hearing about the laser. Now, after two full treatments, her birthmark has gradually faded to a pale pink. "It's astonishing," she says. "No pain, and the treatment took only a matter of minutes. I felt a little warmth, but it went away in about an hour. If you can handle a sunburn, you can handle this."

Carol had test patches treated with the argon, but most of her treatment was done with the newer pulsed tunable-dye laser, which requires no anesthesia. This gentler treatment can be used on children for both port-wine stains and strawberry hemangioma, which looks like a raised port-wine stain. Most hemangiomas disappear by themselves after five to ten years, but this safer laser treatment has made it practical to remove them immediately.

Other skin blemishes involving blood vessels, such as so-called spider veins on the face, can be removed successfully and painlessly with tunable-dye lasers.

"Before lasers, there were no good surgical options for such problems," says Dr. Achauer. "Lasers have really revolutionized the treatment of these types of birthmarks."

Erasing a Memory

We all do things we later regret, but few things are as regrettably permanent as a tattoo—until you include lasers in the picture. Formerly, the best that could be done was a procedure called dermabrasion, which is just as painful as it sounds. Ironically, it often left a negative image of the tattoo. But lasers can remove tattoos with much less scarring and little pain. Just ask Deanna Branch.

Seven years ago, Deanna's shoulder was tattooed with a picture of a heart being pierced by a lightning bolt. Seven months ago, she had it removed with an argon laser. Was she frightened? "No, I just wanted to get rid of it. And my doctor was so enthusiastic about the laser that I believed in it, too."

Deanna's trust was not misplaced. While she still needs a touch-up to remove some remaining pigment, her tattoo is virtually gone. "The skin is a little faded, but there's no scar," she says.

For Women Only

Lasers have a remarkable number of uses in gynecology. The two main reasons for this: the laparoscope and the CO_2 laser.

The laparoscope is one of several long, thin tubes with high-tech attachments that doctors use to look around inside the body. It's snaked into the abdomen through a small surgical cut, and a fiberoptic thread allows the gynecologist to see and examine the ovaries and other important organs without major surgery. The scope can also transport the light of a laser. The great advantage of this combination is that the laser can be used to treat a problem, with only a minimal incision, the moment it's found, rather than waiting for a more extensive second operation.

Two conditions are regularly treated with laser laparoscopy: endometriosis and infertility. Endometriosis is a painful condition in which uterine-like tissue shows up in other parts of the abdomen—in the stomach, intestines, and ovaries—and begins to bleed. Infertility can be caused by endometriosis or by scar tissue on the fallopian tubes and ovaries. In each case, the laser vaporizes the unwanted tissue with virtually no internal bleeding.

The laser is also used externally on the vulva, vagina, and cervix to remove precancerous lesions and warts caused by the papilloma virus. The real advantages of the laser are precision, speed, and minimal scarring, according to Mark A. Rettenmaier, M.D., a gynecologic oncologist at Beckman. Laser treatments cost a few hundred dollars more than conventional therapies, but they seem to be worth the expense.

One promising laser treatment on the horizon: laser hysterectomy. The YAG laser has been used experimentally in a small number of cases to vaporize the lining of the uterus (not to remove the uterus as in conventional hysterectomy). It's less traumatic than a regular hysterectomy but more expensive, and it isn't widely available. Its long-term effects aren't yet known.

Targeting the Ear, Nose, and Throat

If you overuse your voice (as professional singers sometimes do), you can develop tiny polyps on your vocal cords and thus impair your voice, says Roger L. Crumley, M.D., an otolaryngologist (ear, nose, and throat doctor) who is chief of head and neck surgery at UC, Irvine. But polyps and small cancers on the vocal cords can be vaporized with the CO_2 laser. "We've got better control over what we're doing than with a scalpel," says Dr. Crumley. "The laser does all the work."

Edward Hughes is a mechanic who went to Dr. Crumley to have polyps removed. The operation is performed under general anesthesia, and Hughes expected to wake up with a sore throat. "But I had no pain," he says. "In fact, I was supposed to keep quiet for five days, but the minute I woke up, they started asking me questions . . . so I answered them."

Further down in the throat, CO_2 lasers are used to vaporize tumors that obstruct the windpipe. "It's a lifesaving procedure," says Dr. Crumley. "There's no other good way to remove them." And in the nose, lasers are used to destroy polyps caused by allergies. The YAG laser is even used to stop chronic nosebleeds caused by a rare hereditary condition.

The middle ear is another place in which the CO_2 laser is useful. Mastoid disease (any one of several different infections, inflammations, and growths in the middle ear) used to be treated surgically with tiny surgical instruments. The laser is a big improvement.

A brain tumor near the ear (acoustic neuroma) is more

easily removed with the laser because it poses less danger of nerve damage than a scalpel does. And stapedectomy—the removal of a tiny bone in the ear—is now a laser procedure in some institutions. When this bone stops functioning properly, it can cause a 70 percent hearing loss, so the laser literally restores hearing.

The laser has revolutionized treatment in these procedures because it can be manipulated in small cavities without disturbing important, delicate structures around it. Lasers don't necessarily lower costs in most of these operations—primarily because they still must be done in an operating room under general anesthesia—but they do improve the outcome. And that's what *really* counts.

Lasers against Kidney Stones

A nonlaser machine called the lithotripter, which breaks up kidney stones with shock waves, has virtually replaced standard kidney stone surgery. But as pieces of the stones are passed out of the urinary tract, the larger ones can get stuck in the ureter on the way to the bladder. The position of the pelvic bones make further shock wave lithotripsy difficult.

Enter the laser. Pulses of laser energy produce shock waves that break up the stone with little risk of damage to any other part of the body.

Conquering Cancer

Although it's only in clinical trials at Beckman and a few other institutions, a cancer therapy using the laser and a drug called HpD (hematoporphyrin derivative) is showing promise.

Michael W. Berns, Ph.D., director and cofounder of Beckman Laser Institute, says that the procedure works like this: HpD is injected into the body and enters the tumors. Normal tissue expels the drug within 72 hours. Cancer tissue retains it longer. HpD is photodynamic, which means that it initiates a chemical reaction in the cells when stimulated by light. If a laser is beamed at the cancer tissue containing HpD, the drug will kill it.

The Food and Drug Administration (FDA) has approved this therapy for experimental use in lung, bladder, and esophageal cancer.

Scouring Arteries with Light

There's currently only one laser that is FDA approved for clinical use in vascular disease: the hot-tip catheter, which has a metal cap that's heated by laser pulses. The metal cap burns through obstructions (cholesterol or a blood clot) so that a balloon catheter can be used to widen blocked arteries. It was approved for use in the legs in February 1987 and is now available in most major cardiovascular centers.

John Eugene, M.D., a cardiovascular surgeon associated with the Beckman Laser Institute since 1982, has pioneered a procedure that may expand the use of lasers in his field. He developed laser endarterectomy, an operation in which the laser is used to vaporize plaque (accumulated cholesterol) in an artery, then used to weld the artery back together. In a regular endarterectomy, a scalpel is used to remove plaque, then the artery is sewn up. The laser not only leaves a smoother surface inside the artery (discouraging blood clot formation or further plaque buildup), but also seems to close the artery with less trauma. So far, the procedure has been performed on arteries in the legs and the neck. Experiments on the heart are the next step.

CHAPTER 3

Heart Therapies on the Horizon

Drugs that suck fatty deposits off your blood vessels are just one advance due soon.

Fast-breaking developments on several fronts have top heart specialists excited about the near future of heart disease treatment and prevention.
They foresee:

- Accurate models of just how atherosclerosis works— models that experts only dream about now.
- Drugs that suck the fatty deposits right off your artery walls.
- A gadget that lets doctors "see" inside your arteries without surgery.
- Genetic tests that predict your cardiovascular future in your chromosomes.

First Glimpse inside the Artery Walls

The big question puzzling heart researchers has been how high fat levels (high cholesterol) in your blood translate into dangerous plaque on your artery walls. The answer may finally be at hand, if a ground-breaking theory recently announced by California researcher Daniel Steinberg, M.D., proves true.

Dr. Steinberg and his colleagues at the University of California, San Diego, think they have discovered how atherosclerosis actually starts at the cellular level. They started with the theory that white blood cells called macrophages gobble cholesterol-carrying molecules (lipoproteins) inside arterial walls, building up into colonies of

19

bloated cells. That buildup creates fatty streaks inside arteries, later creating an anchor for platelets and debris to cling to. The result is atherosclerotic plaque. And a plaque-occluded artery can easily be plugged by a clot, producing a heart attack in a coronary artery or a stroke in the brain. Until now, researchers couldn't prove this theory because they couldn't induce macrophages to ingest lipoproteins in the laboratory. But by first putting the lipoproteins through a process called oxidation, in effect turning them rancid, Dr. Steinberg created a meal the white blood cells couldn't get enough of. The breakthrough came when the scientists looked into human tissues. "Our laboratory findings were confirmed when we later demonstrated that oxidized lipoproteins really are present inside artery walls," says Dr. Steinberg.

Cardiologists are excited about the implications of Dr. Steinberg's work. They're eager for the results of a Swedish study that may prove the oxidation theory. It involves use of an antioxidant called probucol. "If the Swedish study of probucol is highly positive, it would suggest that a drug that fights atherosclerosis by preventing oxidation of lipoproteins may be a useful adjunct to cholesterol-lowering drugs," predicts Dr. Steinberg.

Who Needs Drugs?

Doctors currently use powerful medications to control very high blood levels of total and LDL (low-density-lipoprotein—the undesirable type) cholesterol that cannot be reduced with dietary changes alone. In five years, experts hope to know whether it is possible, desirable, and safe to use drugs to lower cholesterol enough to reduce existing plaque on artery walls, and perhaps even stop the process at an early stage. Several promising new candidates now being tested are producing dramatic reductions in cholesterol.

Safe cholesterol-lowering drugs will enable doctors to reduce cholesterol to levels they would not be able to achieve by other means. "Right now we have evidence that rigorous reduction of LDL cholesterol prevents further vessel narrowing in people with known vascular disease," says Eugene Passamani, M.D., of the National Heart, Lung, and Blood Institute. "In four to five years we expect to know how much one can safely lower LDL and whether very dramatic reduction results in substantial reversals of atherosclerosis."

"But no matter how advanced drug therapy becomes, we won't use drugs to lower cholesterol unless we have to," adds Robert DiBianco, M.D., of the Washington Adventist Hospital, Takoma Park, Maryland, who expects the use of nutritionists by family doctors to increase. "I foresee more doctors referring their heart patients to dietitians who have the time and training to teach people how to make the necessary dietary changes in their lives."

Invasion of the Noninvasive Devices

So we'll know for sure where our HDL (high-density-lipoprotein—the desirable type) and LDL blood levels should be and have better drugs available to control our bloods fats, but we'll also need better testing devices to diagnose problems and monitor treatment progress.

"The 'holy grail' many of us are searching for is a noninvasive way to monitor permanent changes in arterial plaque resulting from our cholesterol-lowering attempts and other preventive measures," says Dr. Passamani. A *noninvasive* test is one that does not involve inserting a needle through the skin and one that can be repeated. For example, researchers are using a device called B-mode ultrasound to track the progress of atherosclerosis—not in coronary arteries, which are too deep for ultrasound, but in carotid arteries, which are closer to the surface. "By using ultrasound repeatedly over time, one can chart the progression of vascular disease and thereby determine whether various preventive measures actually work," explains Dr. Passamani.

Another contender for "holy grailship" is magnetic resonance imaging (MRI), used today for a variety of deep-tissue applications, such as diagnosing joint injuries. A number of labs are looking at MRI as a way to visualize the coronary arteries themselves without surgery.

Detecting Genetic Risk— Before It's Too Late

You probably know that family history is a major risk factor for heart disease. The problem is, if your father had heart trouble, you could develop the disease while your brother, who smokes, lives until 90 and shows no signs of coronary disease. He may even have high blood pressure and elevated cholesterol levels but still seem the picture of health. What gives?

Like blue eyes, which can be passed on to one child while another's eyes are brown, the tendency toward heart disease is a genetic roll of the dice. But unlike the color of your eyes, cardiac symptoms don't normally show up until middle age or later. If you could know at 20 that you had inherited your father's weakness, you could minimize the danger by avoiding other risk factors, like smoking and obesity, and by getting regular medical checkups to detect early signs of disease.

What would a genetic test look like? According to Dr. Passamani, your doctor would take a blood sample and extract the white blood cells to examine their genetic material. Your chromosomal pattern would then be compared against known "problem" genes. For example, one gene might produce a tendency to develop fatty deposits inside artery walls.

"Research is moving rapidly toward solving the hereditary puzzle," says Dr. Passamani. "But we're handicapped by the complexity of atherosclerosis. Compare it with Huntington's disease, for which we've identified the genetic fault and developed a screening test. Huntington's is caused by one gene, so it's called *monogenic.* Unfortunately, we know that atherosclerosis is *polygenic,* that is, it's caused by multiple genes working in concert. That will make the puzzle harder to solve.

"In five years we may not have the genetic test, but we'll be a lot closer to it. We're working on expanded charting of family trees, so we can look at all family members and predict who has a particularly dangerous or hardy background," he says.

Some Trends Will Continue

"Five years is not a long time in medicine," in the view of Dr. DiBianco. In actual practice, Dr. DiBianco thinks trends, rather than big breakthroughs, will have a more immediate impact on people with and without heart disease. "Therapeutically, I see coronary bypass surgery becoming less common as a first option for men with clogged arteries. Angioplasty, using a balloon catheter to stretch open occluded arteries, is making great strides and becoming a more available alternative to bypass surgery. I see angioplasty used in the future to help delay bypass surgery until a patient has the need for more extensive changes in the blood supply, valves, or muscles of the heart."

Recommended levels for total and LDL cholesterol are likely to remain constant in the next five years, by the way, until the national cholesterol average drops by a significant amount. Experts say *that* development is likely to take longer than five years.

CHAPTER 4

Big Miracles
in Small Packages

Machines smaller than a hair may soon be saving lives.

A machine so small it's invisible to the human eye. What could it possibly do?

Could it send microscopic grinding gears into arteries to clean out atherosclerotic plaque, saving untold numbers of human lives each year? Create artificial organs that function with a precision rivaling the human machine itself? Program pills to deliver and dispense drugs with exquisite accuracy for maximum impact on disease with no damage to healthy tissue?

Well *micromachines* that can do all this and more are just around the corner in research and development, according to a recent National Science Foundation workshop. A new technology unveiled there—called *microdynamics*—has scientists around the country buzzing about the tantalizing possibilities.

Future Wonders

In their report, entitled "Small Machines, Large Opportunities," the researchers describe some medical advances these minimachines may make possible as soon as the turn of the century:

- Lighter and cheaper prosthetic devices, perhaps even artificial organs.
- "Smart pills" with sensors that can detect the surrounding environment and use that information to regulate the drugs they dispense.
- Connectors for repairing damaged blood vessels.
- Individual cell sorters that could count your white blood cells or actually manipulate sperm for artificial insemination.
- A micromechanical ultrasound system that could be mounted on a catheter to give high-resolution, two-dimensional images of damaged tissue inside the body, greatly improving the visuals that guide a physician performing endoscopic surgeries such as arthroscopy.
- Smaller catheters that would allow surgeons to operate inside the body without major surgery, using multiple instruments simultaneously.
- Expansion of catheter-based diagnosis and treatment beyond coronary arteries to areas like gastrointestinal cancers or pancreatic tumors.
- Improvements in the manual dexterity of surgeons themselves, who could use these microfabricated tools to perform more delicate operations, work longer on an operation, and extend their working careers beyond the limits imposed by age-dependent hand steadiness.

• Tiny, artery-clearing cutting devices for use in advanced angioplasty.

Consumer products will also benefit from microdynamics. Impossibly small high-performance audio, video, and computing equipment, as well as amazing animated toys and robots, will become everyday reality.

"Like microelectronics, microdynamics could lead to products as advanced beyond present ones as a compact disc is beyond a long-playing record," says AT&T Bell Laboratories researcher Kaigham Gabriel, Ph.D.

In the Beginning, a Gear

So the microscopic gear the width of a human hair, with a shaft that's one-fifth as wide and teeth the size of red blood cells, is no longer a dream but an idea made real by scientists working at AT&T Bell Laboratories, the Massachusetts Institute of Technology (MIT), and the University of California, Berkeley. Dr. Gabriel says the gear came about when "some of us had the idea that you could build mechanical widgets the same way you build electronic widgets like the printed circuit boards used inside computers."

In microgear construction, layers of two different silicon materials are stacked in the desired shape. One of the materials (silicon oxide) is chemically removed, and what's left is a freestanding working mechanical mechanism made of polysilicon. Incredibly tiny tongs, cranks, levers, and springs can also be manufactured in this manner, and yes, they all really move!

Next, the Motorized Microgadget

"The gears prove that you can build preassembled devices on silicon," says Dr. Gabriel, "but a gear that's just a few molecules thick also needs a Lilliputian motor to drive it." For this pint-sized power plant, Dr. Gabriel and other researchers, such as MIT's Stephen Senturia, Ph.D., plan to harness the free energy of static electricity.

"The static electricity that moves a speck of dust toward

a charged-up sweater is strong enough to power a microscopic gear," says Dr. Gabriel. He says that Richard Muller, Ph.D., a professor of electrical engineering at Berkeley, has already made a miniature gear move with such an electrostatic motor. "The challenge now," says Dr. Gabriel, "is to combine all these elements into a working minimachine."

One of the main obstacles facing researchers is finding a way for our massive human hands to manipulate these microdevices. "They are nearly invisible to the unaided eye," says Dr. Gabriel, "and you can blow them away with a gentle breath."

The scientists also have to determine just how small they can go. "Knowing whether the only limits are the sizes of atoms or whether the limits are slightly higher will be helpful," says Dr. Gabriel.

CHAPTER 5

The Total Cholesterol Story

By Glen C. Griffin, M.D., and William P. Castelli, M.D.

With five kinds of blood cholesterol, it's no wonder the numbers get confusing. Here's your guide to how much of which ones spell trouble.

You may already know your cholesterol numbers, but if you don't, we suggest you find out what they are right away. And why do we say *numbers* instead of *number?* Because there are different kinds of cholesterol and different cholesterol numbers.

Let's start with the single number called *total cholesterol.* You were born with a total cholesterol level of about 70, but as soon as you started eating, it started going up, reaching about 150 by the time you had your first birthday.

After a child's cholesterol level reaches about 150, it usually stays there until he or she is about 17 years old. Then the level starts going up again, often reaching 210 to 220—the average cholesterol level of adults in the United States, Canada, and similar cultures.

Most people around the world don't have cholesterol levels that high, however. People in many parts of the world have total cholesterol levels around 150—and they don't get coronary artery disease. The reason: They don't eat as much saturated fat as most North Americans.

While most adults around the world have cholesterol levels under 150, half of the children in the United States and Canada already have cholesterol levels higher than that.

The problem has been compounded because until recently, many doctors did not become excited about a person's total cholesterol unless it exceeded 300. In the past, some cardiology textbooks said not to worry unless a person's total cholesterol was over 250. But we know from studies like the Framingham Heart Study that most people in our population who suffer a heart attack have total cholesterol levels between 200 and 250.

Much of our knowledge of how cholesterol relates to coronary heart disease comes from studies like the Framingham study. As data from this study show, at virtually any age, the heart attack rate rises 2 percent for each 1 percent rise in total blood cholesterol. This is even true for people over age 65.

The average total cholesterol level of a man in the Framingham Heart Study who had a heart attack in the first 16 years of our study was 244—and now, 30 years later, that level is about 235.

Knowing Your Cholesterols

But total cholesterol isn't the only indicator of risk. You have to consider kinds of cholesterol—or more precisely, ways cholesterol is shuttled about inside your body. So we say there are five kinds of cholesterol—distinguished by the little fat droplets called lipoproteins that transport the cholesterol in your blood.

The largest droplet, or particle, is called a chylomicron. These chylomicrons appear in your blood after you eat fat. The next smaller size particle is called a very-low-density lipoprotein (VLDL). These carry not only cholesterol but also fatty substances known as triglycerides.

Until recently many doctors thought that triglycerides were not very important in relation to heart disease. But you should know that some people with elevated triglycerides are headed for a heart attack, especially if their triglycerides exceed 150 and their HDL cholesterol is less than 40. But hold on. We are getting ahead of our story.

The next smaller particle is the intermediary-density lipoprotein, called IDL. These particles are dangerous if their level becomes elevated, but you probably don't need to worry about these, because few people have this problem.

The next smaller particle is the most dangerous of all because it carries over half the cholesterol in your bloodstream. This is the low-density lipoprotein, or LDL. LDL is bad and is known as the lousy lipoprotein or bad cholesterol!

The four cholesterols we just described (chylomicron, VLDL, IDL, and LDL) are bad for you and tend to collect in your blood vessels. Fortunately there is a fifth cholesterol— and it turns out to be good. This "good" cholesterol is carried by high-density lipoproteins and is therefore called HDL cholesterol. HDL apparently picks up cholesterol from deposits all over the body and brings it back to the liver, where 95 percent of the cholesterol is excreted.

No wonder HDL is known as the good or healthy cholesterol! Research shows that the higher a person's HDL level, the lower the incidence of a heart attack.

Beyond Total Cholesterol

We are now having a campaign in the United States to get everyone to find out their total cholesterol level. The National Heart, Lung, and Blood Institute, part of the National Institutes of Health, has formed a dedicated group called the National Cholesterol Education Program (NCEP) to get the message to the public. The first part of this important message is that everyone needs to know his or her total cholesterol level because high total cholesterol can lead to fat blockages of the arteries (hardening of the arteries). High total cholesterol is anything over the 200 mark we mentioned earlier. (For the NCEP guidelines, see "What to Do about Your Cholesterol Numbers.")

What to Do about Your Cholesterol Numbers

If your total cholesterol falls within these ranges, here are recommendations you should follow, from the National Cholesterol Education Council's summary of recommendations.

Under 200 (desirable): Follow a prudent diet, quit smoking, lose weight if needed, exercise, relax, recheck in five years.

200 to 239 (borderline high): If any two of these risk factors apply to you, see your doctor for an LDL check: male gender, high blood pressure, smoking, heart attacks in the family, HDL less than 35, diabetes mellitus, overweight. If your LDL is under 130, you're considered to be at low risk. If your LDL is over 160, you need a low-saturated-fat, low-cholesterol diet because you are considered to be at high risk.

If you don't have two of the risk factors or don't have a history of clogged arteries, follow a prudent diet, exercise, don't smoke, and have your cholesterols checked annually.

240 or more (high): See your doctor for an LDL check. If your LDL is over 160, you require a low-saturated-fat, low-cholesterol diet because you are considered to be at high risk.

But even though risk generally rises as cholesterol rises, some people with a cholesterol level over 200 are in serious trouble—and some are not. The best way to tell if you are in trouble is to also know your HDL, or "good cholesterol" level, and figure out a simple ratio by dividing the big number, total cholesterol, by the little number, good HDL cholesterol.

For example, if your total cholesterol is 200 and your HDL cholesterol is 50, your ratio is 4 (200 divided by 50), which is very good.

But if your total cholesterol is 210 and your HDL cholesterol is 30, your ratio is 7 (210 divided by 30), which is bad.

Using the same math, if your total cholesterol is 150 and your HDL cholesterol is 43, your ratio is 3.5, which is very good.

An optimal ratio is 3.5, but for starters, we would be quite happy if you and everyone else in North America had a ratio of total cholesterol to HDL cholesterol that was under 4.5. To accomplish this would require that about half the people in North America stop eating so much saturated fat and cholesterol.

From diet and drug research studies, we know that if you lower your blood cholesterol level enough, you can significantly reduce the risk of a heart attack. If you consistently eat a low-saturated-fat and low-cholesterol diet and control your cholesterol levels for a long enough time, regression of the fat plaques may start to occur.

As we said, the best test to judge how you are doing when your cholesterol is over 200 is to check the HDL cholesterol in your blood. Indeed, once your total cholesterol is over 150, you need to know your HDL level because if your ratio of total cholesterol to HDL cholesterol is over 4.5, you are still at an increased risk of having a heart attack.

This is also true of triglycerides. Once they are over 150, you need to get your HDL over 40, or you could be in trouble.

The Two Big LDL Numbers

If your cholesterol is over 240, if you have a cholesterol level between 200 and 239 with two risk factors, or if you already know you have some plugged arteries, your doctor will probably have your LDL cholesterol checked. Then what?

Then two new numbers pertaining to LDL cholesterol will be crucial to you. These are 130 and 160.

If your LDL number is under 130, that's considered a low risk. You will be advised to follow a prudent diet, exercise, and not smoke.

If your LDL is over 160, you will be advised that this is bad, bad, bad! You will be instructed to go on a low-saturated-fat and low-cholesterol diet. You may also find that medications are needed to get your LDL number under 160.

But if you already have cholesterol deposits in your arteries or if you have two of the risk factors, you will be treated with a low-saturated-fat, low-cholesterol diet. If necessary, medications will be prescribed to bring your LDL to under 130.

The Bottom Line

To some, success is getting the LDL under 130. To others, it is getting the ratio of total cholesterol to HDL cholesterol below 4.5.

We know it's better to combine the two standards: Get your ratio under 4.5 and get your LDL cholesterol under 130. Of course, ensuring a good ratio means keeping your total cholesterol under 200. And the key to getting all these numbers where they should be is eating less saturated fat and cholesterol.

Maintaining "good numbers" is one of the biggest steps you and your doctor can take to improve the odds that you don't have a heart attack.

PART II:
NEW STATE-OF-THE-ART
TREATMENTS

Flash Reports

ARTHRITIS DRUG
COMES TO AMERICA

An anti-arthritis drug that's been popular for years everywhere but the United States has received the Food and Drug Administration's stamp of approval. The drug, diclofenac sodium (sold as Voltaren), will be available by prescription for osteoarthritis, rheumatoid arthritis, and ankylosing spondylitis. Its advantage, particularly for older people: It's quickly eliminated from the bloodstream but continues to work in the joint fluid for up to 24 hours, which means it's less likely than other anti-inflammatories to build up to toxic levels.

NEW ULTRASOUND
SAVES SIGHT

A new ultrasound device to treat glaucoma, the disease characterized by high pressure in the eye, has been approved by the Food and Drug Administration. One glaucoma expert believes the treatment could prevent many of the 5,500 cases of blindness the disease causes each year.

Here's how it works: A probe placed over the eye releases pulses of high-intensity sound waves. The waves do two things: They create small pores in the whites of the eye, releasing the built-up fluid that increases pressure. And they decrease the eye's production of fluid. The procedure is painless (a local anesthetic is used), and the usual side effect is temporary inflammation.

The treatment's not for every glaucoma patient, though. Michael E. Yablonski, M.D., chief of the glaucoma service at Cornell University Medical Center, thinks that patients who can't be treated with drugs should turn to laser surgery, which is a more proven procedure than ultrasound at this point. If that fails, ultrasound is the next step. (In certain cases where surgery is known to have a low success rate, ultrasound may be used first.) Dr. Yablonski believes that the new treatment can correct 70 to 75 percent of the glaucoma cases that surgery can't.

HEART ATTACK TREATMENTS TEAM UP

The largest study ever on heart attack victims, involving more than 17,000 worldwide, shows for the first time that *combining* two old, simple treatments substantially reduces heart attack deaths. The treatments are streptokinase (a clot-dissolving drug given intravenously at the hospital) and aspirin (one-half tablet, or 160 milligrams, daily for a month after the attack).

The trick is to work quickly: Using the therapy within 4 hours of the first heart attack symptom decreased chances of death to 53 percent of the odds for patients who didn't get the treatment. But even delayed by 24 hours, the therapy reduced the death rate by an impressive 38 percent, better than any other treatment available currently.

Samuel Z. Goldhaber, one of the study's U.S. coordinators, expects an aspirin-plus-clot-dissolver therapy to become standard quickly.

A sequel to the study is already in the works. This will see if combining aspirin with a different clot-dissolving drug is a slicker ticker treatment.

EXPANDING USES
FOR BALLOONS

Balloon catheterization (or balloon dilation), a procedure commonly used to widen narrowed arteries, is now also being used experimentally in some prostate gland and fallopian tube blockages.

During the procedure, a tiny balloon is inflated at the blockage site, expanding the site without the need for surgery. In the prostate, the technique is most successful in patients who have enlargement of the side lobes. In fallopian tube blockages, it seems to work best on obstructions that occur where the tube joins the uterus.

What is the advantage of balloon catheterization? It's an outpatient procedure that requires only local anesthetic. Its possible disadvantages are that doctors have yet to determine how long results last and that the procedure is not suitable for everyone.

CHAPTER 6

Say Good-Bye
to Gallstones

We now have new ways—and new waves—to rid ourselves of these painful stones.

Some 20 million Americans have gallstones, and until recently the only remedy for this painful problem was surgery. Now, however, you may be able to turn to drugs that dissolve stones or even to experimental sound waves that shatter them. Even more exciting, preliminary evidence suggests for the first time that stones may be preventable.

Most gallstones are formed from bile, a thick, yellow, cholesterol-rich liquid that aids digestion in the small intestine. Bile is produced in your liver and flows out through a tube called the bile duct. Until needed, bile is diverted from the bile duct through a smaller tube, the cystic duct, for storage in your gallbladder. There in your gallbladder, when there's too much cholesterol in the bile, cholesterol somehow clumps together with other substances to create stones.

That's when the anguish often begins. It's also when many people start wondering about a tiny organ that they never thought about before. So here we present some questions that people typically ask about gallstones—and some surprising answers from doctors and scientists across the country:

Q. *I went for medical tests recently and my doctor said he discovered something completely unrelated—gallstones. But I never felt them. How could I have gallstones and not know it?*
A. One-third to one-half of all people who have gallstones don't know it. Most doctors think that if these "silent," or asymptomatic, stones are accidentally discovered, they should be left alone until they cause pain. And the chances of silent stones ever becoming painful are quite small.

Q. *I've had three gallstone attacks in the past two years. They got worse each time. Does this mean the gallstones were getting bigger?*
A. No, not necessarily. Stones do vary in size. The largest reported stone was—ugh!—6.8 inches in diameter, but that is very rare. Most stones are between ⅛ and ¾ inches. These pebble-sized stones cause the majority of painful attacks. When the gallbladder squeezes to release bile, a stone may shoot up and plug the opening of the cystic duct. "The gallbladder becomes an isolated chamber—it squeezes down and tries to empty itself, but bile can't flow out," says Lawrence Way, M.D., professor of surgery at the University of California, San Francisco. The result? Intense pain in the upper abdomen and possibly nausea or vomiting. The pain increases and peaks until,

after several hours, the stone falls back into your gallbladder, ending the attack.

A more serious situation occurs for about 10 to 15 percent of people with symptomatic gallstones. Instead of dropping back into the gallbladder, a stone occasionally travels out of the cystic duct and lodges in the bile duct. Even more rarely, a gallstone actually forms in the bile duct. Any stone that blocks bile flow in the bile duct can cause infection. You're likely to get jaundice. These stones have to be removed.

Q. *Are stones produced continually, like widgets coming out of a factory on a conveyor belt?*
A. It's more like the stones are quarried in batches. Inside the gallbladder, you're likely to find a cluster of stones of one size and a cluster of stones of a markedly different size. But you won't find stones ranging from tiny to large. "The only conclusion is that the onset must occur abruptly, so it's not as if you are in jeopardy of producing stones all the time," says Dr. Way. "But it may be that something happens one day to create little stones, and then they grow."

Q. *I know a lot of women who have gallstones but few men who have them. Is gender a factor in this problem?*
A. Women are three times more prone to gallstones than men. Experts suspect that hormones are involved. Another clue is that taking estrogen or oral contraceptives can increase the amount of cholesterol in bile and thus the chances of having gallstones. (Drugs like clofibrate, a cholesterol-lowering drug, can do the same thing in both men and women.) Also, with each pregnancy, the chance of having gallstones increases.

Q. *My mother had gallstones. Her sister had gallstones. And now I have gallstones, too. Do gallstones run in families?*
A. Yes. There's a definite genetic factor in gallstone development. First-degree relatives (parents, siblings, offspring) of people with gallstones are two to three times more likely to develop gallstones themselves. Also, Native

Americans have the greatest risk of any ethnic group. Almost 75 percent of American Indian women over age 30 have gallstones. Mexican Americans also have more stones, probably because many are descendants of Native Americans.

On top of the genetic influence is the fact that you're more likely to develop gallstones as you age.

Q. *I went on a weight-loss program and lost 30 pounds—and developed gallstones. So did three other women in my group. Was this a coincidence?*

A. Being 20 or more pounds overweight puts you at double or triple risk for gallstones. Paradoxically, losing that weight quickly can also double your risk. Both obesity and rapid weight loss can increase the secretion of cholesterol into your bile.

A 68-person study from Cedars-Sinai Medical Center in Los Angeles, however, gave the first good evidence that gallstones may be preventable during weight loss. Those in a weight-loss group taking ursodiol—a recently approved drug used to dissolve stones—developed no gallstones, while 26 percent in a weight-loss group taking placebos did develop them.

The researchers, however, don't recommend using ursodiol while losing weight until their findings can be confirmed in another study. Also, because they can't predict who will develop gallstones during weight loss, the doctors hesitate to treat everyone. After all, 74 percent of patients in the group that took ursodiol wouldn't have developed stones anyway.

Another possible preventive (not yet recommended) is common aspirin. Preliminary research suggests that aspirin and related compounds may prevent gallstones in obese people during weight loss or halt their recurrence in people who had their stones dissolved with drugs. (Aspirin is thought to inhibit substances that may cause cholesterol to crystallize into stones.)

Eventually both ursodiol and aspirin may help prevent development of stones in Native Americans and others at risk.

Q. *I've had two gallstone attacks in the past year. To be honest, it's not a big problem, but I'm wondering if I should have gallbladder surgery.*

A. If your attacks are mild and occasional, there generally are no health consequences other than pain itself. As long as they stay that way, whether or not you should submit to the knife depends on how much discomfort you're willing to put up with—how painful the attacks are and how much they interfere with daily activities.

Once symptoms begin, however, they're likely to continue and get even worse. And the more often you have attacks, the more likely you are to develop acute pancreatitis or cholecystitis—relatively serious complications that require hospital admission and probably surgery.

Many doctors recommend treating gallstones when convinced that pain is gallbladder related. For people with no serious health problems, surgery is considered the most effective treatment. It's the only way to get rid of stones, pain, and risk of complications for good. Nonsurgery treatments banish existing stones, but the stones often recur within a few years. That's one reason why gallbladder removal is the second most common operation in the United States. If you're otherwise healthy, the procedure is one of the safest. It takes only an hour and requires a four- to five-day hospital stay.

If a stone lodges in your bile duct, however, immediate treatment is necessary. If you're a good surgical risk, a surgeon will probably remove both the stone and your gallbladder. If you're a poor risk, the stone may be removed by sphincterotomy. In this procedure, an endoscope is passed down through the mouth to the intestine. The opening to the bile duct is widened, and the lower end is snipped to remove the stone. "In many cases," says Dr. Way, "somebody who looks pretty sick can have the sphincterotomy and an hour or two later look like a million bucks."

Q. *I don't understand how a gallbladder can just be removed without causing major health problems. Don't I need it?*

A. It's nice to have, but it's not a necessity. Your digestive system works just as well without a gallbladder. Instead of being stored in the gallbladder, bile will simply flow directly from the liver to the small intestines. After your gallbladder's gone, you won't need any special diet or medicine. And cholesterol gallstones will never return.

Q. *I know someone who seemed to have severe gallbladder attacks, so she had her gallbladder removed. But later she still had the same pain. How can this be?*
A. Although ultrasonic pictures can show if you have gallstones, doctors cannot always be certain that the stones are what's causing your pain.

So in some cases, patients with gallstones and pain in the upper abdomen have had their gallbladders removed, only to have the pain persist. The real cause of the pain may be irritable bowel syndrome, ulcers, pancreatitis, or some other abdominal problem.

Q. *I've been diagnosed with gallstones, but the attacks have been mild. Is there any way I can keep them from acting up?*
A. Although controversial, diet may have a place in treating symptomatic gallstones. In humans, it's not yet clear what role diet plays in the formation of gallstones. But fatty foods are known to stimulate gallbladder contractions, and presumably these contractions shoot stones into the duct, causing a gallstone attack.

So consider a diet with only 25 percent of your calories coming from fat (generally 40 to 50 grams of fat per day). This means you should minimize added fats—salad dressings, gravy, butter, or margarine. Stick to low-fat cheese and use skim milk instead of whole milk. Eat only lean meats—no more than 6 to 7 ounces a day.

Consuming smaller, more frequent meals may also help limit gallbladder contractions and gallstone attacks.

"There is a large individual response to diet, and I think the best rule of thumb is to do what works for you," says Karen Miller-Kovach, a registered dietitian who is spokesperson for the American Dietetic Association. "If you have gallstones and find that larger or fatty meals bother you, then cutting back is worth trying."

And all the other health benefits you reap from a low-fat diet make it an even better bet.

Q. *I've been told that I can flush gallstones from my system by fasting for three days and then drinking a mug of olive oil and lemon juice. Anything to it?*

A. Olive oil—an old folk remedy—may flush stones, but it isn't considered effective or safe. The fat in the olive oil could cause the gallbladder to contract and push through extremely small stones. But it's just as likely that somewhat larger stones would shoot out into the duct and become stuck.

Q. *I have severe gallstone attacks, but I don't want to have surgery. Can't the stones just be zapped with lasers?*

A. Well, not lasers, but there are other high-tech techniques under experimentation. One is lithotripsy. This is the use of shock waves to shatter stones. (Drugs are then taken to dissolve remaining fragments.) It works like this: A water-filled cushion is held against your abdomen while a spark plug discharges, causing the water to suddenly evaporate and generate a shock wave that disintegrates the stones. The procedure is repeated for up to two hours. You can undergo lithotripsy only if you have a small number of stones with a minimal amount of calcium in them—which means only about one in five people with gallstones is qualified. Lithotripsy is effective only 70 to 80 percent of the time.

Another experimental method involves inserting a tube into the gallbladder and pumping in a chemical solvent to dissolve stones in a few hours. This can be used for any number of stones, but they must contain no calcium. Both lithotripsy and this chemical infusion are now done at only a handful of medical centers around the country. The main drawback is that with both techniques—and unlike surgery—gallstones often recur.

Q. *What about this new drug, ursodiol, that dissolves gallstones? Why isn't everyone using it instead of surgery?*

A. Ursodiol (brand name Actigall) was approved for general use in late 1988. Another oral drug, Chenix, was developed several years ago but was little used because it often caused liver damage. Ursodiol does not. Its only side effect is temporary diarrhea.

Drug therapy for gallstones is limited to people with small cholesterol stones who, because of health reasons, are at greater risk of complications from surgery. It may also be a good option for qualified people who don't want surgery.

Ursodiol has its drawbacks, though. It can take up to two years to dissolve stones and is effective only 50 to 75 percent of the time. Treatments cost $1,500 a year, and half the time, stones return after you stop taking the drug. (Compare this with once-and-done $10,000 gallbladder surgery.)

CHAPTER 7

A How-to-Take- Common-Drugs Guide

By Joe and Theresa Graedon

What you eat along with a pill can help or hinder its absorption.

Oil and water don't mix. That you know. But do you know which prescription medications don't mix well with food? Over the years there have been occasional sightings (like UFOs) in the literature of food-drug interactions, but nobody seemed to pay much attention. A few drugs were known to be highly irritating to the stomach, so doctors generally prescribed these to be taken "at meals." Other than that, there wasn't a whole lot of talk about food doing much to or for drugs.

Things are slowly changing.

The growing study of pharmacokinetics (the real measure of what happens to drugs after they enter your body) has led to an appreciation that a lot of things have an influence on how a drug gets absorbed and used (or not used) by the body. Among those factors, food turns out to play a significant role for many medications. In some cases, foods enhance a drug's absorption. But more often, some foods delay the entry of drugs into the bloodstream or prevent it entirely.

Food Interference

For example, many antibiotics—such as ampicillin or penicillin (Amcill, Omnipen, Pentids, Pfizerpen, Polycillin, Principen, Totacillin, and many other brand names)—are less effective if taken with food. Acidic drinks, such as wine, soda pop, coffee, and fruit juice, may also be a problem.

The exact formulation of the drug can make a big difference, too. Erythromycin comes in various guises, including erythromycin stearate (Bristamycin, E-Mycin, Erypar, Erythrocin, Ethril, Pfizer E, and Wyamycin S), erythromycin estolate (Ilosone), and erythromycin ethylsuccinate (E.E.S., EryPed, and Pediamycin).

All of these are broad-spectrum antibiotics often prescribed for a variety of infections, including those in the ear, throat, and urinary and reproductive tracts. Erythromycin stearate is less effective if taken with food.

But studies have shown that the other two forms are absorbed at least as well (if not better) with meals as on an empty stomach. Acidic beverages are also a problem with erythromycin, so don't wash your pills down with orange juice or cola.

Take your tetracycline (Achromycin, Cyclopar, Sumycin, Terramycin, Tetrex, and others) with meals and as little as half of it may get to work. Make that a meal containing milk products—or take a calcium supplement at the same time—and you can reduce that effectiveness to about 10 percent. You'd be paying a buck to get ten cents' worth of help. Worse than that, ten cents' worth is perhaps worse than no help at all, because it can mean the elimination of the weakling bacteria and the enhanced growth of the more resistant strains. You can wind up with an infection that's incredibly resistant to cure.

Laxatives containing bisacodyl (Carter's Little Pills, Dulcolax, Fleet, Theralax) shouldn't be taken with dairy products, either. They are designed to dissolve and go to work in the intestine. But when you wash them down with milk, they tend to dissolve in the stomach and cause irritation.

In general, calcium carbonate supplements (Biocal, Calcitrel, Cal-Sup, Caltrate 600, Os-Cal, Suplical, Tums, and others) should be taken with meals. (This is especially true for older people, who often have lower-than-normal levels of stomach acid—a condition that can drastically cut absorption of calcium carbonate.) But still you have to watch for specific foods that can interfere with absorption.

Fruits and vegetables that contain oxalates, such as spinach, rhubarb, beets, green beans, gooseberries, and blackberries, should not be eaten within two hours of taking a calcium pill. That goes double for whole wheat bread. Not only does it contain oxalates, it is also rich in absorption-reducing phytic acid, as are other whole grains like oats, barley, and rye. Black beans, almonds, limas, brown rice, soybeans, and peanuts are also full of phytate. Imagine the woman who sits down to a healthy breakfast of oatmeal, shredded wheat, or bran cereal and then pops down her calcium supplement. Less of her calcium is likely to make its way into her body and go to work.

People with an underactive thyroid gland are often put on thyroid supplements, such as Cytomel, Euthroid, Levothroid, Synthroid, and Thyrolar. Certain foods, however, can interfere with the action of the thyroid gland and compromise an already sluggish system. Do not overdo on cabbage, kale, kohlrabi, cauliflower, rutabagas, turnips, brussels sprouts, and soybean products like tofu.

People who have had blood clots (thrombophlebitis, pulmonary embolism, heart attack, or stroke) are often prescribed an anticoagulant, such as Coumadin (warfarin). It works to thin the blood by blocking the action of vitamin K. If you eat large quantities of foods high in this nutrient, you could undo the benefits of your medicine and end up in the hospital with another clot. It's ironic that many of these foods are especially healthy and are often recommended for low-fat diets. Don't pig out on cauliflower, brussels sprouts, spinach, cabbage, broccoli, green beans, peas, leafy greens (turnip, mustard, collard), beef liver, soybean oil, and green tea. But don't eliminate all these foods, either, because you need some vitamin K to prevent hemorrhaging. To be on the safe side, have periodic blood tests to make sure your blood is clotting properly.

Gout can cause episodes of excruciating pain when uric acid crystals build up in joints, especially in the big toe. Drugs that are commonly prescribed to control uric acid levels include Zyloprim and Lopurin (allopurinol), Benemid (probenecid), and Colbenemid (probenecid and colchicine). For these drugs to work most efficiently with the least risk of kidney stones, people taking them should avoid foods high in purines—anchovies, sweetbreads, brains, kidney, liver, gravies, scallops, herring, mackerel, sardines, spinach, broth (beef and chicken), lentils, and other legumes.

Red Alert

Certain drugs interact with particular foods in a much more alarming way. Isoniazid is the drug of choice for treating tuberculosis in older people. But besides working better on an empty stomach, isoniazid could provoke a disastrous reaction if you happened to take it with certain foods high in an amino acid called tyramine, especially pickled herring, Stilton cheese, Camembert cheese, Cheddar cheese, Emmentaler cheese, brick cheese, Roquefort cheese, Gruyère cheese, salted dried fish (like salt herring), mozzarella cheese, meat extract (gravy base, Marmite, and others), Parmesan cheese, beef liver (stored), Romano cheese, Brie cheese, chicken liver (stored), provolone cheese, processed cheese, avocado, and Chianti and other red wines.

This list is arranged with the foods highest in tyramine at the beginning. If someone were to indulge or overindulge in one of these foods while taking isoniazid or the antidepressants Marplan (isocarboxazid), Nardil (phenelzine), or Parnate (tranylcypromine), the result could be a very dangerous reaction, pushing blood pressure through the ceiling.

Isoniazid has another little-known quirk. It would be wise to stay away from fish, especially tuna and skipjack,

Drugs That Work Better without Food

The following drugs are known to be adversely affected by food. It'd be nice to say that this list is complete, but it isn't. If your drug is not included, it may mean that food does not interfere with it. But more likely, it means there's not much research available.

Acetaminophen (Anacin-3, Datril, Tylenol, Cosprin)
Ampicillin (Amcill, Omnipen, Supen)
APAP
Aspirin, coated (A.S.A. Enseals, Easprin, Ecotrin)
Bisacodyl (Dulcolax, Fleet)
Calcium citrate (Citracal)
Calcium phosphate (Posture)
Cefaclor (Ceclor)
Erythromycin stearate (E-Mycin, Ethril)
Furosemide (Lasix)
Isoniazid (Laniazid, P-I-N Forte)
Levodopa (Dopar, Larodopa)
Magnesium hydroxide (milk of magnesia)
Mineral oil
Nafcillin (Unipen)
Oxacillin
Penicillamine (Cuprimine, Depen)
Penicillin G (Bicillin)
Penicillin V (Nadopen-V)
Penicillin VK (Beepen-VK, Pen-Vee-K)
Procainamide
Propantheline bromide (Norpanth)
Rifampin (Rifadin)
Tetracycline HCl (Cycline, NorTet, Robitet, Sumycin, Tetrex)

(continued)

Drugs That Work Better without Food—Continued

Theophylline (Theo-24)
Tolmetin (Tolectin)
Trimethoprim-sulfamethoxazole (Bactrim, Septra)

   Note: Medicines such as the heart drugs procainamide and quinidine, aspirin and other arthritis remedies, iron supplements, the Parkinson's disease drug levodopa, and others may need to be taken with meals to reduce stomach irritation, even though food may limit absorption. A drug that causes irritation for one person may not cause problems for another. Any side effects should be discussed with your physician or pharmacist.

while on this medication. This interaction may not be as life threatening as if one were eating pickled herring, but a person going through the histamine response that would result could easily feel as if he or she were dying!

Playing It Safe

The list could go on and on, but by now you have begun to get the idea that food and drug interactions can be extremely important. Consult "Drugs That Work Better without Food" for a list of some of the drugs that interact with foods, and also press your doctor and pharmacist to give you some definite information about the subject whenever they hand you a prescription or fill it. (If you are told the medicine must be taken on an empty stomach, generally you should swallow it at least an hour before meals or two hours after. Following it with a full glass of water is usually a good idea.) If these professionals can't supply you with the information, ask them to find out about any food interactions of the drug by asking the drug company directly.
   Perhaps if pharmaceutical manufacturers get enough

inquiries from doctors and pharmacists on behalf of enough patients, they will gather the information we all need.

CHAPTER 8

Don't Put Up With Incontinence

Simple changes in diet and bathroom habits are sometimes all that's needed for a cure.

The problem began for Sally, a nurse and an aerobics instructor, when she was in her late twenties. During jumping jacks or jogging, small amounts of urine would leak. Her make-do solution: sanitary napkins.

A few years later, after her first child was born, the problem worsened. "When I went back to aerobics, I would wear two maxi-pads and soak them both." Finally, she sought medical treatment.

Sally's doctor recommended a new surgical treatment. And within a few days, Sally was back to leading aerobics classes—with no more wetness.

Sally was hardly alone with her problem. The National Institutes of Health estimate that at least ten million adult Americans experience urinary incontinence, the involuntary loss of urine, ranging from the occasional leakage of a few drops to complete loss of control.

Urinary incontinence is twice as common in women as in men, and older people are more susceptible. However, incontinence is no more a normal part of aging than chest pains or diabetes, says Neil M. Resnick, M.D., director of the continence center at Brigham and Women's Hospital in Boston. "It's not inevitable and it's not irreversible. It can be a symptom of an underlying disorder that warrants medical attention, so you should see a physician, but for the vast majority of people, it can be treated." Sometimes, as in Sally's case, a new and relatively minor surgical procedure can cure the problem. But often treatment involves simple changes in diet and bathroom habits, or practicing special exercises.

Of course, cure depends on diagnosis. But more than half of incontinent people have never had their problem evaluated. Women are especially shy about broaching the subject, says incontinence expert Katherine Jeter, Ed.D., E.T. (enterostomal therapist), founder of the self-help organization Help for Incontinent People (HIP). "Men will drip once or twice and they're in the doctor's office," says Dr. Jeter. "Women will drip for nine years and not tell anyone. Maybe they figure this is part of the curse of womanhood. Then, too, it is very hard for a woman to look a male physician in the eye and say, 'I just started wetting my pants.' "

Experts agree that shame can be one of the most devastating consequences of urinary incontinence. "I call incontinence a social disease," says urologist Robert Schlesinger, M.D., who directs the continence clinic at the Faulkner Hospital in Boston. "People will go to almost any extent to adjust their lives to it. We had one woman who didn't go out of her house for three years because she was so ashamed."

It needn't be that way. The National Institute on Aging and other branches of the National Institutes of Health have put incontinence near the top of their agendas. More physicians are learning about the problem. "There is now a clear message that people should not be stigmatized by it," says Dr. Jeter. "Nearly everybody can be made better or cured."

What Is Urinary Incontinence?

Incontinence is not a disease. It is a symptom of an underlying condition affecting the urinary system. The urinary system includes two kidneys, two ureters, the bladder, the urethra, and the sphincter muscles. The kidneys remove waste products from the blood and produce urine.

Urine flows through the ureters to the bladder, where it is stored until it exits the body through the tubelike urethra. The sphincter is a muscle that wraps around the urethra and, like a purse string, controls its opening and closing. In men, the prostate gland is also wrapped around part of the urethra. The pelvic area is crisscrossed with muscles that hold these organs in position for proper function.

What can go wrong? Often incontinence is triggered by a temporary and curable problem such as a urinary tract infection or medication that can loosen the grip of the sphincter muscle. The pelvic muscles can be weakened or damaged by obesity, childbirth, injury, or surgery. In men, prostatic enlargement or prostate surgery can affect the urethra and the sphincter. A host of diseases, such as diabetes, multiple sclerosis, spinal cord injury, and Parkinson's disease, can damage the nerve pathways between bladder and brain.

Although old age doesn't cause incontinence, the changes that come with aging make older people more vulnerable. With age, the bladder shrinks, sphincter strength declines, and the pelvic muscles can lose tone. In women, declining hormonal levels can lead to inflammation and atrophy of the urethra. Add an illness or injury, and urine loss can result.

Doctors describe four common patterns of incontinence, each with many possible causes:

- Stress incontinence (which has nothing to do with psychological stress) is when a cough, a sneeze, a laugh, bending over, lifting, running, or any slight abdominal pressure triggers leakage. It can be related to the muscles supporting the bladder and urethra; if they're weak or damaged, those organs sag and the sphincter cannot shut properly.
- Urge incontinence is when people feel a compelling need to go and immediately lose their urine. Local irritation or infection can trigger the involuntary bladder contractions that cause leakage.
- Overflow incontinence is when a person doesn't feel any urge to void, so the bladder fills to capacity and the excess spills over. Primary causes are diabetes and, in

men, a bladder blockage due to an enlarged prostate gland.

• Reflex incontinence refers to the complete loss of bladder control because the brain never registers the need to void. Among the causes are spinal cord injuries and stroke.

Tracing the Leak

If you have incontinence, it's very important to consult a physician. "It could be a sign that something else is seriously wrong. Usually that 'something' can be easily identified and readily fixed," says Dr. Resnick.

A physician will take a medical history and perform a physical examination, including a pelvic and rectal examination, blood tests, and urinalysis. You may be asked to urinate into a funnel-like contraption that measures urine output. Less comfortable tests may require insertion of a catheter (small tube) through the urethra into the bladder to measure bladder function. Other, specialized tests may be required as well.

Behavioral Therapy

Treatment, of course, will depend on the cause of incontinence. The following three behavioral therapies can reduce incontinence for many people, and cure it for some.

Pelvic muscle exercises. Ever hear of Kegels? They're the contract-and-release pelvic muscle exercises developed in the late 1940s by Arnold Kegel, M.D., that are usually used to help women with stress incontinence. They are usually recommended for women during and after pregnancy. But experts say that they can reduce and possibly prevent some forms of incontinence in people of all ages.

Unfortunately, not everyone gets the hang of them right away, and they do require frequent practice if the benefits are to be sustained (see "How to Do Pelvic Muscle Exercises"). Various studies have reported benefits for 30 to 90 percent of women who practice them correctly.

Biofeedback. "Biofeedback is used to teach somebody to do a Kegel and understand what it is they're expected

How to Do
Pelvic Muscle Exercises

Keeping the sling of muscles around the urinary system taut and in good shape is a key to continence, says Katherine Jeter, Ed.D., E.T., director of Help for Incontinent People (HIP). If you practice regularly, you may experience improvement in a few weeks or months. (Be sure to consult your physician.) These exercises, called Kegels, may even prevent incontinence. Here are HIP's instructions.

To identify the muscles you'll be exercising, first, without tensing the muscles of your legs, buttocks, or abdomen, imagine you are trying to hold back a bowel movement by tightening the ring of muscles around the anus. Do this exercise only until you identify the back part of the pelvic muscles.

Next, when you're passing urine, try to stop the flow, then restart it. This will help you identify the front part of the pelvic floor. (Women: Another way to think of this is that you are trying to grip a slipping tampon.)

Now you're ready for the complete exercise. Working from back to front, tighten the muscles while counting to four slowly, then release them. Do this for two minutes, at least three times daily.

You can do this exercise anywhere, sitting or standing, while watching TV or waiting for a bus. It's important not to tighten the abdominal, thigh, or buttocks muscles. Tightening the abdomen, in fact, can push urine out.

If you're not certain whether you're doing the exercise correctly, talk to your physician or nurse, who can check you while you're doing it or use a biofeedback apparatus to teach you.

to do," says Dr. Schlesinger. People can be taught to contract the sphincter, as in a Kegel, and to relax the abdomen and bladder in order to prevent urine from being pushed out.

How does biofeedback work? It's like a computer game. A small sensor is placed into the vagina of a woman or the rectum of a man. It's linked to a computer screen or other output device. Patients are instructed to contract or relax the appropriate muscles; at the same time, they can watch rising or falling lines on the screen that show them how they're doing. "One lady told me, 'This is better than playing Atari!' " says Dr. Jeter. Studies indicate that biofeedback training can cure 20 percent and improve another 30 percent of patients with stress and/or urge incontinence.

Habit training. First, people are instructed to void at regular short intervals—such as hourly—during the day. Over a few weeks, they increase the interval, up to four hours. The technique is used primarily for stress and urge incontinence. Physicians can't explain why habit training helps. "We don't know whether it truly retrains the bladder to function normally or whether it trains the brain to cope with a persistent bladder dysfunction," says Dr. Resnick.

Medical Treatment

There are many people whose incontinence can be completely cured simply by switching or removing a medication, says Dr. Resnick. Certain prescription medicines, including some of the drugs prescribed for high blood pressure, can trigger bladder control problems. So can some over-the-counter drugs like diuretics, decongestants, multicomponent cold medicines, sleeping pills, and diet pills, which stimulate the involuntary nervous system that affects the bladder.

On the other hand, the following medications and medical treatments can bring about needed relief.

Incontinence drugs. For urge and reflex incontinence, physicians sometimes prescribe medications that relax the bladder and, in so doing, block the involuntary contractions that lead to urge incontinence. Unfortunately, these medications may cause side effects such as dry mouth, blurred vision, constipation, or more serious problems. "It takes teamwork between cooperative patients and physicians to get the exact dosage to achieve the best results with a minimum of side effects," says Dr. Jeter.

Estrogen therapy. Some postmenopausal women with incontinence have benefited from estrogen therapy, since the lower part of the urethra is affected by the same hormones as the vagina.

Suspension surgery. Although in most cases surgery should be a last resort, surgical techniques for correcting stress incontinence in women are better than ever. In the past, surgical correction of a sagging bladder and urethra required opening the entire abdomen; recovery could take weeks and the operation was not considered appropriate for many elderly people.

Today, doctors usually perform "suspensions" for stress incontinence, to return the urethra to its normal well-supported position. A suspension involves two stitches sewn between the abdomen and the inside of the vagina; the stitches act as slings to hold up the urethra. The procedure can be completed in 45 to 60 minutes with a minimum of anesthesia; it requires only a short hospital stay and has a high success rate. (This is the surgery that helped Sally, the aerobics instructor.) Even very old patients tolerate it well.

Other surgery. Prostate surgery, tumor removal, or repair of previous surgical damage may be required. (Incidentally, hysterectomy is not an appropriate treatment for incontinence, except in very rare instances when the condition is associated with a uterine abnormality.)

The artificial urinary sphincter. When all else fails, a silicone system that mimics the body's sphincter mechanism can help some people. Among them are young people with spina bifida and some men whose radical prostate surgery has resulted in incontinence.

Where to Get Help

Not every health care provider is equally qualified to treat urinary incontinence. "You're looking for someone with compassion—someone who will not dismiss your complaint, but rather show a keen interest in resolving it with you," says Dr. Jeter. Start with your family physician, gynecologist, geriatrician, or urologist. Many nurses have developed an expertise in incontinence, including those who work in urology, enterostomal therapy, rehabilitation, and geriatrics. They can do initial assessment, referral, and teaching of behavioral techniques, says Dr. Jeter. Finally, check to see whether there's an incontinence clinic in your area. There's a growing number across the country.

For more information, contact Help for Incontinent People (HIP), P.O. Box 544P, Union, SC 29379. HIP offers self-help information and patient advice (send a stamped, self-addressed, business-sized envelope—$1 donation optional). Or contact the Simon Foundation for Continence, P.O. Box 835, Wilmette, IL 60091, which offers information and has support groups across the country and internationally. (Call toll-free, 1-800-23-SIMON, or send a self-addressed, stamped, business-sized envelope.)

CHAPTER 9

Update on Intermittent Claudication

Painful leg cramps are one symptom of this disease, a sign that the arteries there are partially blocked.

It happens like this: You're out for a stroll (minding your own business) when suddenly—ouch!—your calf cramps up like a knot on a rope, making even one more step unthinkable. You rest for a couple of minutes until the pain subsides. Mobile again, you get just about as far as before, when . . . zowie! You didn't know they made cramps this bad! Just what's eating your leg, anyway?

Intermittent claudication, probably. To most of us, that

just means occasional lameness. But to a doctor, it also may mean that a lifetime of bad habits is catching up with you.

Intermittent claudication is a sign that your leg arteries are partially blocked. When you walk, your leg muscles don't get enough blood, gradually become oxygen deprived, and . . . gotcha! A cramp. The malady is caused by the same type of blockage that the coronary (heart) arteries suffer: atherosclerosis, in which plaques of fatty deposits form inside the vessels. So the same things that cause atherosclerosis, such as smoking and high cholesterol levels, can cause intermittent claudication (also called peripheral vascular disease).

Assessing the Problem

This is no time to dwell on past mistakes, though. Luckily, there's plenty you can do right now to stop the problem from getting worse, to increase the distance you can walk without pain, and perhaps even to reverse the damage. And should the need arise, medical science has come up with new and safer ways to remove the blockages.

While the symptoms mentioned above are a pretty good indication of claudication, they're not the only ones. The pain could be in your foot, thigh, hip, or buttocks. And it could feel more like an ache or tired feeling. But since other diseases can masquerade behind these signs, and claudication itself is a serious disorder that can lead to amputation, the first step (once your leg unkinks) should be in the direction of your doctor.

"A diagnosis could be made with a fair degree of reliability based on your symptoms alone," says Daniel Levy, M.D., director of the cardiology laboratory at the Framingham Heart Study.

But your doctor won't stop there. He will check the pulses in your leg arteries and listen for signs of constriction and will also check the blood pressure in your lower leg. (If it's much lower than in your arm, there's probably some blockage.) And you may be recommended for an ultrasound test, which can give a better idea of the degree of atherosclerosis.

"But," says Dr. Levy, "an angiogram, where dye is injected into the vessels and x-rays are taken to determine the exact location of the blockages, should not be done unless your doctor feels you may need surgery or another procedure, because of the risk of complications."

Your doctor should also check for signs of heart disease. "The incidence of coronary artery disease [CAD] in patients who have peripheral vascular disease [PVD] is about 75 to 80 percent," says Robert Ginsburg, M.D., director of the Center for Interventional Vascular Therapy at Stanford Medical Center. "So if you have PVD, the odds are that you have CAD."

That may be true even if you are not having any symptoms. "People who have intermittent claudication tend not to be able to exercise much, and it's exercise that tends to bring on symptoms of coronary disease," says Dr. Levy. "So there may be a masking phenomenon, where the claudication masks the severity of the coronary disease."

Your doctor will also check for a high cholesterol level, high blood pressure, and diabetes, because they all contribute to the problem.

Once all the information is in, your doctor can decide on the best course of action. "The important thing is that the person making that judgment should be an internist or general practitioner who can refer you to a vascular surgeon if necessary," says Dr. Ginsburg.

Treat Yourself to Relief

The first line of defense for most patients is not miracle drugs or laser surgery. It's eliminating the risk factors that caused the problem in the first place and taking some positive steps to keep the legs in top form. "About 80 percent of people diagnosed with claudication will stay stable, 5 percent will improve, and 15 percent will deteriorate," says Mark Creager, M.D., director of the Noninvasive Vascular Laboratory at Brigham and Women's Hospital in Boston and assistant professor of medicine at Harvard Medical School.

The problem is, you don't know which of those groups

you fall into (although people with diabetes and those who continue to smoke tend to do the worst). That's why it makes sense to do everything you can.

Quit smoking. Doctors aren't sure how cigarettes cause atherosclerosis, but they do know that it's the number one risk factor for claudication. "Patients who claudicate are almost universally cigarette smokers," says Dr. Ginsburg. "I don't think I've ever seen a claudication patient in my life (except for those with diabetes) who did not smoke at some time. The most crucial thing is for them to stop smoking. It helps dramatically."

Start walking. Surprisingly, one of the best remedies for intermittent claudication is "the hair of the dog that bit you"—walking! How can the thing that hurts help? "When you walk until the skeletal muscle in the legs becomes oxygen deprived, it stimulates an autoregulatory process in the body to increase blood flow to the legs," says Dr. Ginsburg. "The body releases local hormones and vaso-active agents that open up the small 'collateral' leg muscle vessels that have been dormant."

These newly opened vessels take over some of the job of the clogged ones. Pain is lessened, and over a period of three to six months, you will be able to walk farther. "You probably won't be able to run a marathon," says Dr. Ginsburg, "but many people go from being house-ridden to being able to shop."

In addition, the extra circulation brings with it the white blood cells that keep infection—the main cause of amputation—at bay. None of these good things will happen if you don't quit smoking, though: Nicotine causes the collateral vessels to remain closed, Dr. Ginsburg says.

The trick is to walk to the point of discomfort, rest, then resume your walk. Dr. Creager recommends continuing this for half an hour, one to three times a day. And don't worry: Evoking the pain isn't dangerous. It's just that if you push too far, your muscles may get weak and precipitate a fall.

Note: Here again, it's important to see your doctor before you bet all your marbles on a walking cure. The reason: If the artery blockage is above the thigh, exercise won't help.

There won't be enough blood coming through to help develop collaterals. Your doctor can determine the blockage location.

Other benefits of walking: It makes you feel better, helps you lose weight and control diabetes better, and increases cardiovascular fitness. In fact, almost any kind of exercise—swimming, bicycling, or whatever—also has these advantages and so can be good for people with intermittent claudication, says Dr. Creager.

Pamper your feet. Since cold can cause blood vessels to constrict and diminish blood flow, patients in northern climes should take extra care to keep their feet and legs warm.

Everyone with claudication, especially diabetics, should take steps to prevent infection. Keep toenails properly trimmed straight across (see a podiatrist, if necessary) to avoid ingrown toenails. Inspect your feet daily for cracks, calluses, corns, and ulcers, and seek treatment by a podiatrist if necessary. Avoid constricting garters. Wear only comfortable, wide-toed shoes—no sandals, and no barefoot strolls. Keep feet clean and moisturize dry skin.

Lose weight. If you're obese, losing weight can help take the strain off a vascular system that's already taxed to the max.

Avoid or control diabetes. Maintaining your normal weight may also help you avoid diabetes. If you already have the disorder, controlling it is crucial.

Reduce your cholesterol level. Doctors know that reducing a high blood cholesterol level by eating a low-fat, low-cholesterol diet helps keep artery blockages from getting worse. And some preliminary studies suggest that aggressive cholesterol reduction may even reverse peripheral atherosclerosis to some degree. That approach looks promising, says Dr. Levy, although there is no conclusive evidence yet.

Control your blood pressure. Again, keeping your blood pressure as close to normal as possible helps prevent claudication and probably slows its progression. Salt restriction, exercise, relaxation techniques, and medication are some of the tools for lowering blood pressure. Discuss the condition with your doctor.

No Drugs to Turn To

All of that may seem like a lot of work, but unfortunately, there is no magic bullet that can wipe away a lifetime of the disease. "In general, drug therapy does not improve claudication," says Dr. Creager. Dr. Ginsburg agrees. "We are testing a whole variety of new agents in randomized, double-blind, placebo-controlled trials here at Stanford to try to answer this question," he says. "So far we have not found an agent that you can demonstrate scientifically improves exercise time or increases blood flow to the legs."

And although there have been some reports that vitamin E or certain chelating agents might be helpful, "no studies have proven they are efficacious," says Dr. Creager.

Dr. Ginsburg does make use of one "wonder drug," however, even though there is no conclusive evidence that it helps. "We recommend that our patients take one aspirin tablet a day," he says. "It's based on experience with carotid artery disease and heart disease, not any solid data on the legs, per se. But it probably prevents further platelet deposition [elements of plaque] and progression of the disease."

You shouldn't try this aspirin regimen without consulting your physician, though, since it may cause serious side effects in certain people.

The Surgical Alternative

Even with the best intentions, conservative therapy may not do the trick, and in some cases a medical procedure to remove the blockage may be necessary. If you are a letter carrier, for example, and painful walking interferes with your work as well as your enjoyment of life, you may be a candidate. If you are having pain while sitting still, the disease has progressed past the point where other measures can help. Or if your leg is in jeopardy from an infection that will not heal, more extensive measures are in order.

In the past, you'd automatically be on track for a bypass procedure, where one of your own veins or a synthetic graft would be used to route blood around the blockage.

But no more. Doctors are perfecting new techniques that appear to be preferable in many cases. One that is catching on like wildfire is called balloon angioplasty. It's the same procedure doctors have been using to open up blocked coronary arteries. A catheter (tube) is inserted into the artery, and a balloon is inflated at the point of the blockage to open it up.

"At Stanford, we use a lot of investigational devices, but the balloon is used in about 80 percent of the procedures," says Dr. Ginsburg. "We also use other mechanical devices, as well as lasers. The bottom line is that in the majority of patients who have need for a procedure, we can open up the blockages by a nonsurgical technique. Most of the time the patients can get in and out of the hospital in one or two days, compared with one to three weeks for a bypass procedure."

Dr. Ginsburg says that angioplasty done in the arteries above the thigh has about a 75 percent five-year patency rate—that is, three-quarters of the patients still have open arteries after five years. A comparable bypass, which is done with a synthetic graft, is 98 percent patent after five years. However, the bypass has a 5 percent rate of complications or death, while the risk is almost 0 percent for angioplasty.

In the lower part of the leg, the procedures are roughly equal in patency rate (55 percent) after three years. But again, angioplasty is much easier on the patient and costs about one-third as much, Dr. Ginsburg says. And you can always do it again. Once your veins are used for a bypass, however, they're unavailable for later use. "The problem is that many patients also have coronary artery disease and may need those veins for coronary bypass surgery later on," says Dr. Ginsburg. "That's why the best thing to do is nothing. Stop smoking and walk. Second, if you're really having problems, have angioplasty. And third, only if all else fails, have a bypass procedure."

Other last-ditch efforts include sympathectomy and endarterectomy. In sympathectomy, following a bypass for advanced disease, the doctor may opt to cut the nerves that allow the blood vessels to constrict in response to cold. (This procedure also cuts the pain fibers, which can bring welcome relief at this point). In endarterectomy, the surgeon makes an incision in the vessel and tries to mechanically scoop out the plaque. "Although it gives you an immediately good response," says Dr. Ginsburg, "it stimulates exaggerated regrowth. Basically, it gums up real fast—in about a year."

The point is, no one need reach the stage where those procedures must be considered, because intermittent claudication is a preventable disease. "Since its causes are largely determined by modifiable risk factors, its principle method of prevention is simply one of cardiovascular disease prevention: blood pressure control, avoiding smoking, cholesterol reduction, and vigorous diabetes control," says Dr. Levy. If we take those preventive measures, intermittent claudication won't be so common in the future.

CHAPTER 10

Fighting Dry-Eye Syndrome

Learn the facts about causes and treatment of this annoying—and potentially dangerous—condition.

Dry eyes. It doesn't sound like much of a problem, does it? But for over nine million people in this country who suffer from chronic dry eyes, it is cause for tears. If inadequately treated, chronic dryness can damage the cornea. In extreme cases, it leads to loss of sight.

Fortunately, the problem rarely progresses to that stage. Treatment for many cases of dry eyes, chronic or not, is simple and relatively inexpensive. And while there's no once-and-done cure for people with certain dry-eye syndromes, there's been a surge of research activity on a number of fronts—with very promising results.

Pinpointing the Causes

Dry eyes aren't unusual, and they don't always indicate that something is wrong. "Some people produce a lot of tears; some don't. It's a natural variation, just like some people are 6'8" and some are 4'8"," says Jay Krachmer, M.D., professor of ophthalmology at the University of Iowa and director of the Iowa Lions Cornea Center. Of course, if you have a lower level of tear production, your eyes are going to be more susceptible to irritation. But there are several pathological causes of dry eyes (or, as scientists call it, keratoconjunctivitis sicca). Most involve either a decrease in tear production or an increase in tear evaporation. Here are the main culprits.

Growing older. One of the most common instigators of dry-eye problems is Father Time himself. As we get older, all our glands—including the tear-producing lacrimal glands—slow down. That doesn't mean everyone over 50 suffers from dry eyes. Some people feel a marked change, but not everyone is bothered by it. Others have more serious problems: chronic dryness that causes pain, blurriness, or a gritty feeling. Older women are more likely than men to have noticeable problems with dry eyes. (The ratio is an overwhelming ten women to every man.) Several scientists suspect a hormonal link related to menopause, but research is still quite preliminary.

Environmental evaporators. When tear production is low but adequate, everything is fine. But there are environmental factors that can hasten the evaporation of tears, pushing marginal tear producers into a deficit or virtually bankrupting people with chronic dry-eye problems.

An extremely hot, arid climate can dry out your eyes. Wind can do the same thing. Dry winter winds are especially nasty, as any skier knows.

Indoor heating is another eye-drying winter hazard. By January or February, air in most buildings in northern climates is annoyingly low in moisture. The summer provides no break, either. Air-conditioning makes dry eyes a year-round indoor problem for some people. And video-display terminals can cause dry eyes—not through any sort of eye-frying radiation, but because of the user's intense concentration. It's well known that we blink less often when reading or staring at a screen (TV as well as VDT). Blinking restores the tear film over your eyes. Looking away for a bit—taking conscious "blink breaks"—is a good idea for people who work with VDTs or have other jobs requiring close visual concentration for long periods of time.

Eyelid and blinking abnormalities. If the eyelid is turned in (with eyelashes touching the eye) or out, or has an irregular margin, then the eye may not close completely, hastening tear evaporation. Eyelid abnormalities are not uncommon as we get older. Tear evaporation can also be hastened by problems with the blinking reflex, which can be interrupted by nerve abnormalities, Bell's palsy, or complications of surgery in the eye area.

Medicinal side effects. Many common prescription and nonprescription drugs can cause eye dryness. Some of the broader categories include antihistamines, beta-blockers, decongestants, diuretics, oral contraceptives, sleeping medications, tranquilizers, and tricyclic antidepressants. Check with your doctor or pharmacist if you suspect a medication-related problem.

Illness. Certain medical conditions can cause dry-eye problems. A thyroid condition known as Hashimoto's disease, for example, and a hereditary disorder known as Riley-Day syndrome can both cause inadequate tear production.

Eyelid damage. The meibomian (*my-BOW-me-an*) glands, located along the edge of the eyelids, produce a lipid (liquid fat) outer layer that slows the evaporation of the watery tear layer below. Local infection or inflammation of the eyelid, known as blepharitis (*bleh-far-EYE-tiss*), can alter the composition of the lipid layer enough to allow increased evaporation. This problem is associated with a number of general skin conditions, including acne rosacea, eczema, and psoriasis. It is quite common.

Sjogren's syndrome. Some people who have dry-eye problems also suffer from a drying of other glands, notably in the mouth and vagina. They may also have swelling of the joints, a feeling of general malaise, and a number of other seemingly unrelated symptoms (anemia, kidney problems, and others). All this can add up to a diagnosis of Sjogren's syndrome, a disorder that affects about one million people in this country.

Sjogren's syndrome is an autoimmune disease, like rheumatoid arthritis. In each, some unknown factor causes the immune system to attack certain parts of the body as if they were foreign invaders. In arthritis, it's the lining of the joints; in Sjogren's, it's primarily the tear-producing lacrimal glands. Infection-fighting white blood cells called lymphocytes attack the glands, causing them to lose much of their ability to function.

As in most autoimmune diseases, women far outnumber men among Sjogren's patients. (The disease affects about nine women for every man.) While Sjogren's can strike at any age, two groups are at greater-than-average risk: women in their thirties and forties who have rheumatoid arthritis, lupus, or a similar chronic disease; and women in their sixties and seventies. About half of all cases of Sjogren's accompany a clinically diagnosed case of rheumatoid arthritis or one of the other rheumatic diseases.

Right now there's no cure for Sjogren's syndrome. At present, treatment consists of easing the symptoms. Some people can function quite well with Sjogren's. Others are much more restricted. "Sjogren's is not usually a life-threatening disease, but it is a lifestyle-threatening disease," says Elaine K. Harris, president and founder of the Sjogren's Syndrome Foundation. Research into the cause of Sjogren's and other autoimmune diseases provides the greatest hope for better treatments—and perhaps even a cure.

Fighting Dryness

For people with Sjogren's and other long-term dry-eye problems, treatment is an ongoing process. The good news: It's a very successful process in many cases.

The type and intensity of treatment are determined not by the cause but by the severity of the dryness. Mild problems can be controlled with ordinary tear-replacement drops. Moderate dryness calls for greater use of the drops in conjunction with various tear-sparing gadgets, such as moisture-chamber glasses. Severe dryness can be treated with all of the above, with surgery as a last resort.

Tear-replacement drops. Also known as artificial tears, these drops are the mainstay of therapy for most people with dry eyes. There are about 30 brands on the market. Most of them are a mixture of saline solution and a "film-forming" substance, such as polyvinyl alcohol or synthetic cellulose. Though polyvinyl alcohol doesn't sound like something you'd want in your eye, it and the other ingredients are perfectly safe.

Doctors often recommend that patients try several brands to see which works best for them. If problems develop with one, you can always switch.

For mild cases of dry eye, most physicians recommend one drop in each eye three or four times a day. This should be done whether or not the eyes feel dry, since prevention is the watchword of all chronic conditions.

Don't use most brands more than five times per day because they contain chemical preservatives to kill bacteria. If you overuse the drops, the preservatives can build up to a toxic concentration and start killing cells on the surface of the eye. Possibly the least-irritating preservative currently in use is sorbic acid.

For moderate to severe cases of dry eye, sufferers use special preservative-free drops about once an hour—for some people, every 15 minutes! As of this writing, two brands of preservative-free artificial tears are available without a prescription: Refresh and Ocu-Tears. There are also special preservative-free formulations that dry-eye specialists can make up, but they're available only by prescription.

A caution: Artificial-tear formulas are quite distinct from anti-redness eyedrops. Use of the latter can relieve some symptoms of dry eyes by constricting blood vessels on the eye's surface. But continued use of anti-redness drops can cause a rebound effect, in which the blood vessels dilate and the eye gets redder. Overuse can lead to serious problems.

Overnight ointments. Even when the lids are closed, eyes can dry out. To prevent overnight problems, several combination tear-replacement/moisture-sealing ointments are on the market for use without a prescription. Most contain petrolatum and mineral oil, with various other ingredients.

Of course, the individual response to these ointments varies. Some people with moderate to severe dry-eye problems find them quite helpful. Others think they're messy and not very effective. It really is a try-it-and-see proposition.

Lacrisert. This is the brand name of the only tear-replacement product that comes in solid form. Shaped like an oblong pellet, Lacrisert is a cellulose-based product that dissolves over the course of a day. The pellet is placed under the lower lid. As it dissolves, it makes the tear film thicker and more viscous. Many people use Lacrisert along with artificial tears.

Lacrisert is available by prescription only. It is probably best for people with moderate dry-eye problems, as people with severe problems find the pellet rather irritating. Some people find that Lacrisert makes their tears too sticky, leaving a discharge on their lashes or blurring their vision.

Antibiotics. People with dry eyes associated with blepharitis can often be helped by treating the underlying inflammation with oral doses of tetracycline. This antibiotic takes two to three weeks to work and should be continued for several weeks thereafter. Blepharitis can recur, but it is relatively easy to control. Extra attention to eyelid hygiene, including warm-washcloth compresses and careful cleaning of the lids, can help prevent further problems.

Moisture-chamber glasses. These work like swimming goggles, except they keep moisture in. The glasses have plastic sides around each lens, forming an airtight chamber. As tears evaporate, the air inside each chamber becomes slightly more humid. This retards further tear evaporation and provides a comfortable, moist atmosphere.

Although they don't sound overly attractive, moisture-chamber glasses can be cosmetically acceptable. The glasses are manufactured with and without prescription lenses.

Dry-eye contact lenses. For people with dry eyes, contact lenses are usually a luxury they must do without. But in a very small percentage of cases, so-called bandage lenses are used to decrease discomfort by keeping the lid from rubbing against the eye. Like regular contacts, these lenses are available only by prescription.

Punctal occlusion. This is a fancy name for plugging up the duct that drains tears out of the eye. The punctal ducts can be closed temporarily or permanently. Temporary closing, or occlusion, is done with tiny plugs that are inserted in the punctal ducts. To test this therapy, doctors sometimes implant plugs made of collagen, a natural substance that dissolves in a few days. If the occlusion seems to help keep the eyes moist, the doctor can implant silicone plugs that won't dissolve. The plugs can pop out, though, and they're not easy to put back in. Still, if the eye has too much tearing, the plugs can be removed without problems.

Permanent occlusion is serious business, and is done only in the most severe cases. It's usually done with a cautery needle: The punctal opening is burned shut. The procedure can also be done with a laser—often at much greater expense. The operation is reversible, but it's not easy. Tiny tubes are implanted in the ducts to keep them open while the surrounding tissue heals.

Surgical options. For people with eyelid abnormalities, corrective surgery can help. Sometimes the problem can be completely corrected. Sometimes symptoms improve, but eyedrops or other therapies are still necessary. As with any surgery, there can be complications, such as infection and scarring. Always get a second opinion before you agree to an operation.

For people with severe Sjogren's syndrome, a form of eyelid surgery called lateral tarsorrhaphy can help preserve moisture. The outer edges of the eyelids are sewn together, reducing the exposed eyeball surface by as much as one-third. The low level of tear production may then be more effective, but that doesn't mean the need for eyedrops is eliminated.

Hope for the Future

Right now scientists and doctors are investigating a variety of products new and old that may turn out to offer help for dry-eye sufferers.

Tear-gland saver. Plaquenil is an anti-inflammatory prescription drug that's normally used to treat malaria. Researchers at Scripps Clinic and Research Foundation are currently testing oral doses of the drug in Sjogren's patients. "In the early stages of Sjogren's, any anti-inflammatory drug may help save the lacrimal glands," says Mitchell H. Friedlaender, M.D., an ophthalmologist at Scripps who's involved in Sjogren's research. "Plaquenil is one anti-inflammatory that people can be given for a long time without many complications."

In one preliminary study, ten Sjogren's patients were given 200 milligrams of Plaquenil every day for one year. Compared to ten Sjogren's patients who received no treatment, all of the Plaquenil group showed significantly reduced autoantibody levels. Further trials are needed, however, before Plaquenil's true value can be assessed.

New preservative-free tear formula. Healon is the brand name of hyaluronic acid, a liquid originally derived from the collagen in rooster combs. Normally, it's injected into the eye to protect and maintain the shape of the cornea during cataract surgery. But a surgeon in Florida got the idea to dilute Healon with saline to make a preservative-free artificial-tear formula. "Many of our patients think it's more soothing than commercial drops," says Vincent P. deLuise, M.D., a Connecticut ophthalmologist who's using the mixture.

Although it isn't yet marketed to the public, some ophthalmologists make Healon drops on request. The main problem is the expense: from $80 to $100 per bottle. Not everyone finds Healon to be significantly better than much cheaper drops. Before Healon becomes a widespread therapy, its claim to superiority must be verified in scientific tests—and its price must plummet.

Eye-healing tears. Fibronectin is a component of human plasma that concentrates at wound sites, seemingly to stimulate healing. Lately, a California company has been isolating fibronectin out of donor plasma (screened for AIDS and hepatitis) and testing it as an eye-healing artificial tear. It promotes a healthful bonding of cells on the exterior surface of the eye. Preliminary results suggest that fibronectin may decrease symptoms associated with dry eyes and reduce damage to eye cells. This data has encouraged the researchers to proceed with a full-scale, double-blind clinical trial. If fibronectin lives up to its promise, it could be useful in a whole spectrum of eye diseases.

Potential tear-gland stimulator. Cyclosporine is an immunosuppressive drug used to prevent the body from rejecting a transplanted organ. A veterinarian at the University of Georgia, in Athens, was the first to test cyclosporine eye drops on dogs with dry eyes. In these tests, tear production in the dogs increased four to five times. And a preliminary study on 12 people at the University of Glasgow, in Scotland, was encouraging. Now, researchers at the Massachusetts Eye and Ear Institute, in Boston, have begun a clinical trial in humans.

At first, it was thought that the immunosuppressive drug counteracted a Sjogren's-like reaction in the dogs. "But we found that it works as well on dogs that don't have any evidence of an autoimmune problem," says Renee L. Kaswan, D.V.M., the veterinarian who pioneered this treatment. Another plus: The amount of cyclosporine used in the drops is 100 times less than the amount used to cause immune suppression throughout the body or that causes any of the other side effects associated with this drug in organ-transplant recipients. The real test will be the results of the human trials, but researchers are optimistic.

Estrogen replacement therapy. In some documented cases, estrogen replacement therapy (ERT) seemed to improve dry-eye symptoms in a few women with estrogen deficiency. The nature of estrogen's therapeutic action in other cases is untested at this time. Some researchers are looking into other hormonal cures as well. All experts agree, though, that the possible effect on dry eyes is only one of many factors to consider in any decision to try ERT.

CHAPTER 11

Put a Stop
to Sinusitis

Here's a quick review of diet, lifestyle, and drug approaches to this frustrating problem.

You wake up at dawn with pounding pain in your head—everywhere, it seems: Your eyes, your nose, your forehead, even your teeth hurt. Your nose is so stuffed up you'd need a Roto-Rooter to unplug it, and thick, vile-tasting fluid keeps dripping down the back of your throat.

A cold turned killer? Close. What you've probably got is sinusitis—inflammation and usually infection of one or more of the eight small cavities within your head called the paranasal sinuses. Anywhere from 30 to 50 million Americans suffer this problem, making sinusitis one of the five most common health complaints in the country.

"Sinusitis is simply an inflammation of the membranes lining the sinuses that can interfere with normal drainage," says J. R. B. Hutchinson, M.D., president of the American Academy of Otolaryngic Allergy.

Sound simple? That's because it is. The big question: Why does such a simple condition cause so many problems?

The mucus produced in our sinuses normally flushes out germs and debris that might otherwise cause infection. When the sinuses become inflamed, drainage stops. When drainage is interrupted for any reason, problems can develop. Sometimes the structure of the nose itself is partly to blame.

"All the sinuses drain into one small nasal area with an outlet about the size of the open tip of a ballpoint pen," explains Richard Mabry, M.D., clinical professor of otolaryngology at the University of Texas Southwestern Medical Center in Dallas. "The nose is very easily plugged up, and when that happens, the trapped fluid becomes the perfect medium for bacterial growth, usually leading to infection."

The congestion of severe sinusitis creates pressure around the eyes and forehead as well as pain in and around the sinuses. Sinusitis can also be accompanied by mild fever and thick discharge from the nose and down the back of the throat—the infamous postnasal drip.

Liquid Protection

Produced in your nose and sinuses, mucus actually contains substances that attack and kill marauding bacteria that happen to land in your respiratory tract.

In a typical day, your body produces about a quart of this key fluid, most of which you swallow without noticing. But when sinusitis hits, the mucus thickens. "People may think they are producing more mucus than usual, but what changes is not so much the volume as its thickness," says Dr. Hutchinson.

Postnasal drip can actually be a good sign: It means your sinuses are draining, which is important in defeating the infection. It can also be useful in diagnosing sinusitis, according to Lee E. Smith, M.D., assistant clinical professor in the Department of Otolaryngology/Head and Neck Surgery at the University of West Virginia. If you've got an allergy or just a cold, the mucus will usually be relatively clear and free flowing, explains Dr. Smith. If you've got sinusitis from a bacterial infection, the discharge will change from clear and runny to a thicker consistency that looks more yellow or greenish.

How do you tell a bad cold from sinusitis? The key distinction is the course of the infection, and that takes some time to develop. "A cold normally starts to get better after about 72 hours," explains Dr. Mabry. "It may drag on for a week, but most of us notice improvement starting around the third day. Sinusitis is the exact opposite: It gets worse after two or three days and continues to worsen."

The message here: If your cold gets worse after three days or you notice a key symptom of sinusitis—increased pain, fever, or a change in nasal discharge—see your doctor immediately.

The Big Three

The causes of sinusitis are just as varied as its symptoms, since essentially anything that produces inflammation in the nose can generate sinusitis. But according to Dr. Mabry, most cases are caused by one of three factors: allergies, structural abnormalities within the nose, or environmental irritants.

Allergies. Allergic symptoms can very closely mimic sinusitis: Your nose is so stuffed up you can't breathe. But with allergies, even when your nose starts running, your sinuses may still drain. Problems begin when allergic congestion blocks drainage from the sinus cavities, actually causing sinusitis.

"The medical history of people who repeatedly come down with sinusitis may not show any clues that an allergy is involved. And often you can't find any indication of a structural abnormality. I find that cases like this are strong indicators to look for an underlying allergy," Dr. Hutchinson says.

Structural abnormalities. This generally means just one thing—a deviated septum, usually diagnosed through visual examination of the nose or by x-ray.

The septum is the cartilage-and-bone wall that separates the two air passages in your nose. Deviated simply means it's crooked. When the septum is crooked, one of the air passages is narrower than the other, and that can lead to blockages.

"This condition is very common," says Dr. Hutchinson. "It's usually the result of a trauma—a fist fight, an automobile accident, or a sports injury, such as a catcher missing the ball and getting hit in the face.

"What patients notice most is that they have trouble breathing through one nostril or that one side of the nose gets congested whenever they lie down," adds Dr. Hutchinson. "This is one of the most common causes of chronic sinusitis, since the path of drainage is blocked."

Environmental irritants. "Pollution is a tremendously important factor in sinusitis," Dr. Smith says. Common pollutants include ozone, associated with automobile and industrial exhausts, and that nefarious nemesis of the airborne traveler—tobacco smoke.

"Tobacco's probably the worst offender," says Dr. Smith. "Hot smoke loaded with tar—it's hard to imagine a worse combination." But again, anything that irritates the nose, be it fumes from the local paint factory or your neighbor's backyard barbecue, can bring on sinusitis.

Climate and geography play major roles in environmental sinusitis. The wetter the climate in your part of the country, the more likely you are to encounter the pollens and other foliage-linked irritants that can cause sinusitis. Valleys can act as natural traps for pollutants and pollens, but if you live by the ocean, your risk is lower: The endless breezes sweep air clean.

"I hardly ever saw a case of sinusitis when I worked at Stanford University in California," Dr. Smith says. "I was absolutely astounded at how many I encountered when I moved to West Virginia, and I think climate and geography are chiefly responsible. Molds, pollens, and pollutants seem to affect people more severely here."

Preventing Sinusitis

There's really no way to shield yourself perfectly against sinusitis. But there's a lot you can do to make your armor less vulnerable:

- Stay away from smoke. If you smoke, stop. If you live with smokers, ask them to do it outside.
- Minimize dust, pollen, and pollution. Keep your house clean to minimize dust in the air. Avoid the outdoors during peak pollution hours—morning and evening rush hours. Keeping the air conditioner on during allergy season may help if you remember to check the filter regularly to make sure it doesn't harbor any mold. Change your filter often. Negative-ion generators have also helped in some cases by removing small particles from the air.
- Humidify the air. "Keeping the air between 45 and 65 percent humidity is really important, especially in the winter," says Dr. Smith. The reason: A dry nose is vulnerable to infection, and humidity can keep yours from doing an imitation of the Sahara. Make sure to

clean your humidifier regularly to check the growth of mildew or mold.

● Drink lots of fluids. One of the most effective ways to prevent infection is to keep the mucus flowing. It won't if you're dehydrated, so make a point of drinking several glasses of water per day and getting plenty of other fluids, such as soup.

● Avoid alcohol. Those fluids you're drinking should not include alcohol. A single night's consumption can mean major misery the next morning, in the form of rebound vasodilation: The blood vessels swell. Then, as the alcohol leaves your system, they shrink—but swell back up again the next morning. The consequences are more swelling, less drainage, greater pain, more risk of infection.

Plugging the Drip

If it's already too late for preventive measures, here are some tips on clearing your clogged, throbbing head.

Use drugs wisely. Treatment for allergy-related chronic sinusitis usually consists of decongestants to permit easier breathing and keep the sinuses draining properly. Your doctor may prescribe antibiotics to treat infection, which is usually caused by staph or strep bacteria frequently present in the nose.

Over-the-counter decongestants are fine, but don't abuse them. "Don't exceed the limit on the bottle," warns Dr. Hutchinson. "You can actually end up with more inflammation instead of less if you do."

Don't try antihistamines, Dr. Mabry cautions: "Antihistamines reduce swelling and let you breathe a little easier, but they also dry up the nose and thicken the mucus— exactly the opposite of what you want to do. Drainage is what you want, not dryness."

Ask your doctor about surgery. If you've got a deviated septum and a history of sinus problems, it makes sense to fix the problem once and for all. Treatment for this kind of sinusitis means correcting the deviation—an outpatient surgical procedure that requires about a week or two for full recovery.

If the idea of surgery intimidates you, weigh it against all those years of pain and misery. Besides, surgical treatment has become highly effective and is getting better all the time. In fact, increasing use of the endoscope, a fiberoptic device for looking inside the nose, now makes surgery more precise than ever and leads to quicker recovery times. The endoscope, which the surgeon uses to guide tiny surgical tools, lets physicians first look at exactly what they want to operate on and then remove it without disturbing surrounding tissues.

"Between 70 and 80 percent of all the patients I've performed endoscopic surgery on showed major improvements, and no one got worse," says Dr. Smith.

Don't forget: No improvement after three days means it's time to see your doctor. The treatment is usually antibiotics, sometimes steroids, or at worst, surgery. Failing to treat sinusitis could lead to much more serious disorders. Untreated sinusitis can lead to serious multiple-bacteria infections that cross over into the brain itself. So do your best to prevent it, and failing that, seek treatment early.

CHAPTER 12

Free Yourself From UTIs

Antibiotics treat urinary tract infections, but they won't stop recurrence. For that you need preventive strategies.

Burning, frequent urination, painful spasms, and occasional bloody urine—these are the all-too-familiar symptoms of urinary tract infections (UTIs). UTIs are caused by bacteria from the vagina or intestinal tract that migrate up the urethra (urine tube) into the urinary tract, where they multiply within 24 to 48 hours and cause infection. Women are particularly susceptible to UTIs because their short urethra allows bacteria to enter the bladder easily. In cases where UTI-like symptoms are caused by sexually transmitted agents such as chlamydia, gonorrhea, or the herpes virus, men are equally susceptible.

Treating What You've Got

UTIs are usually diagnosed by urinalysis and treated with high doses of antibiotics taken for one to three days. If you have a UTI, it's important that your doctor perform a pelvic exam to check for sexually transmitted diseases, especially if you're nonmonogamous or have a new sex partner. Insist on a test for chlamydia. Recurrent urinary tract infections require diagnosis by culture and antibiotics for seven to ten days.

Most doctors also advise women with UTIs to drink eight glasses of water daily for several days and to refrain from vaginal intercourse until symptoms disappear.

Self-care may be effective for women with mild UTIs:

- Drink large amounts of water.
- Urinate frequently.
- Avoid vaginal intercourse until symptoms disappear. However, if symptoms do not subside within a day or two, see a health professional.

Pregnant women with UTIs should not attempt self-care, as they are more likely to develop kidney infections with nausea, vomiting, chills, high fever, and the need for hospitalization. Kidney infections in pregnant women have been associated with premature delivery and babies with low birth weights.

Preventing Recurrence

You *can* prevent painful urinary tract infections. Here's how:

- Both partners should wash their genitals and hands before sexual activity. If frequent infections are a problem, use an antibacterial soap or Betadine skin cleanser.
- Avoid transporting bacteria from the anal area into the vagina. Wipe from front to back and thoroughly wash anything that has been in contact with the anus before touching the vagina.
- Drink a glass of water and be sure to urinate as soon as possible after intercourse. Then drink six to eight glasses of water during the next few days, and urinate frequently to keep any bacteria from multiplying in your bladder.
- If you suffer from frequent UTIs, avoid intercourse during menstrual flow, when blood can be pushed into the urethra and encourage bacterial growth.
- Diaphragm users frequently suffer urinary tract infections because the diaphragm rim may press on the urethra and prevent complete emptying of the bladder. You may need to switch to a smaller size diaphragm or to a cervical cap or condoms.
- Birth control pill users also frequently develop bladder infections. You may need to switch to another form of birth control.
- Catheters commonly used after delivery and during or after surgery often cause infection. Tell your doctor you want to avoid catheterization if at all possible. Request privacy and adequate time in the hospital so you can urinate on your own.
- Avoid intercourse with any new partner who may have a sexually transmitted disease. If you engage in sex, be sure to use condoms and spermicide. If symptoms develop following sex with a new partner, request a urinalysis and gonorrhea and chlamydia tests.
- If you suffer from recurrent UTIs, try taking one antibiotic tablet after sex. Talk with your clinician to ensure you're using the appropriate antibiotic.
- If you suffer frequent UTIs and have a supportive physician, you may be able to save time and money through self-diagnosis. There are simple, safe, dip-and-read tests on the market that allow early detection of UTI. (One brand is Chemstrip LN, which includes 100 test strips

per vial, with instructions and color-change chart. It is available from the Self-Care Catalog, P.O. Box 130, Manderville, LA   70470.) At the first sign of symptoms, dip a test strip into a urine sample. A color change indicates UTI. Then call your physician and get a prescription by phone—without an office visit.

• If you continue to suffer from symptoms and your doctor says all signs of infection have been eradicated from your bladder or vagina, try the following: Cut all caffeine and alcohol out of your diet. (Both increase urine flow and may irritate the bladder.) Avoid intercourse for two or three weeks. (Masturbation is okay.) Get a referral to a urologist. Chinese medicine may also help: See a specialist in herbal medicine and acupuncture.

CHAPTER 13

Make Sure Your "Pressure" Medicine's Not Squeezing Your Heart

---

While decreasing blood pressure, some antihypertension medications actually raise blood cholesterol. Check out your type, then check with your doctor.

In North America, more than 50 million people have high blood pressure. Many take prescription drugs to keep their pressure down. But recent studies suggest that these pills sometimes do more harm than good.

Taking some antihypertensive medications is like driving your car with one foot on the gas and the other on the brake. These drugs decrease blood pressure, but some *increase* blood cholesterol. And researchers believe that for every 1 percent increase in blood cholesterol, heart attack risk goes up 2 percent.

If your doctor wants to put you on any blood pressure medicine, check to make sure that it does not increase cholesterol. If you take any blood pressure medication that raises cholesterol, have a complete blood cholesterol evaluation, including total cholesterol, high-density lipoprotein (HDL), low-density lipoprotein (LDL), and HDL-to-LDL ratio. Have these tests repeated at a later date to make sure your cholesterol level has not increased. In some cities you can get these tests for free if you donate blood to the Red Cross.

The newly discovered connection between blood pressure medications and increased cholesterol levels may explain why some people who take these drugs have trouble getting their cholesterol down. Sad to say, many high blood pressure sufferers are also treated with cholesterol-lowering drugs. Such medications are often very expensive and frequently have unpleasant side effects of their own. For some people, the drugs are essential because of a genetic disposition, but for others, high cholesterol may have been triggered by their blood pressure pills.

Control without Cholesterol Complications

Luckily, a number of effective antihypertensives don't increase cholesterol. These include calcium channel blockers (Adalat, Calan, Cardizem, Isoptin, and Procardia), the angiotensin converting enzyme (ACE) inhibitors (Capoten, Prinivil, and Vasotec), the vasodilator Apresoline, and the alpha-blocker prazosin (Minipress).

ACE inhibitors are revolutionizing the treatment of hypertension because they don't cause the fatigue, forgetfulness, sexual side effects, or depression that are common with beta-blockers and some other antihypertensive medications. But they have to be used very carefully. If your kidney function is not normal, they may be quite toxic. Thus, before taking these drugs, make sure the doctor does a creatinine clearance test. And avoid potassium-containing salt substitutes while taking the ACE inhibitors. With these drugs, too much potassium can be just as dangerous as too little.

On the horizon, Minipress looms as a healthful alternative. This drug actually appears to *decrease* cholesterol levels. Minipress may also turn out to be useful for prostate problems. According to preliminary research reports, Minipress relaxes the smooth muscle in the prostate that makes urination difficult for some men with prostate problems. Minipress may thus help postpone the need for prostate surgery. If early studies are borne out by later research, this could be an important boon to the millions of older men who experience diminished urine flow due to overgrowth of the prostate gland.

If you have high blood pressure and need to be on drugs, discuss the cholesterol issue with your doctor. Know your options and make sure you keep track of your own cholesterol levels.

CHAPTER 14

Open Your Eyes to New Eyewear Advances

Today's eyeglasses and contact lenses let us see better and look better.

Eyeglasses were invented way back in the thirteenth century, just about the time that shining armor was going out of style. But it took more than 400 years for someone to figure out that hooking them onto the ears was the best way to hold them on the face!

Luckily, eyeglass technology has progressed somewhat faster in recent times. Now, in addition to having their hands free for other tasks, eyeglass wearers can set their sights on a new breed of bifocals, on lenses adapted to their favorite sport, and specs that make their job easier. New, ultralightweight lenses take a load off their nose, and antireflection coatings make nighttime driving a breeze. Lenses that filter ultraviolet light may even help prevent cataracts and other eye diseases.

The news in vision aids doesn't stop at glasses, though. Contact lenses are now being used to reshape the eye, actually improving vision. New materials are being used to make the healthiest contacts ever, and disposable contacts are now available. And coming soon to an optometrist near you—lenses that treat eye diseases.

For a closer look at the latest developments in eyewear and how they can benefit you, read on.

New Help for the After-40 Problem

Presbyopia sounds like an exotic disease, but it's really just a commonplace vision problem. Though it starts at about age 10, most people don't begin to experience the effects until they're in their forties. By age 50, virtually everyone has it.

Simply stated, presbyopia is a disorder that results in a gradual decline in the ability of the eye lens to focus on nearby objects (hence the arm's-length approach to reading in so many over forty).

Bifocals (and trifocals) have been used to alleviate this problem for years. The lenses have segments with added power (typically in the lower half) for reading or other close work. What's new is the advancement in an improved version called progressive addition lenses. "Instead of an abrupt change between the segments for distance and near vision, these lenses have a gradual increase in power as the wearer looks downward," says James Sheedy, O.D., Ph.D., associate clinical professor at the University of California, Berkeley, School of Optometry. The result more closely resembles natural good vision, and people can use the middle portion of the lens to spot objects at in-between distances. Some people also find these new lenses easier to adapt to. And since there is no visible line between segments on the lens, only your optometrist knows for sure.

For people who prefer the uncluttered vision that contact lenses afford, there are now bifocal contacts available in hard, soft, and rigid gas-permeable lenses. "They're similar to regular bifocals, except that they sit on the eye," says Wayne Cannon, O.D., chairman of the contact lens section of the American Optometric Association. "You see at distance through the top part of the lens. But when you look down at something close by, the lens moves up so the segment for near vision is over the pupil."

Although it usually takes more skill to fit them properly and more time to adjust to them, most people can wear bifocal contacts successfully.

The New Focus on Sun Protection

With more and more people learning that overexposure to sunlight may do permanent damage to the eyes, demand has grown dramatically for lenses that can protect eyes from ultraviolet (UV) light.

"Short-term overexposure to UV unquestionably causes a temporary inflammation of the front of the eye, resulting in redness, itchiness, and a gritty feeling," says Dr. Sheedy. "But of more concern is the growing evidence that long-term exposure to UV could contribute to cataract formation. There's also some evidence that it might contribute to some retinal disorders."

So many optometrists are advocating UV-protecting glasses, especially for anybody at high risk:

- People who've had cataract surgery (in which the eye's lens is removed, exposing the retina).
- People who spend most of the day outdoors or who work near snow or sand (which reflect more UV into the eyes).
- People who live at high altitude (where there is a 15 percent increase in UV for every 3,000 feet in altitude).

- People who live nearer the equator (such as those in the southern United States).
- People who regularly take prescription drugs that increase sensitivity to UV light (some oral contraceptives, tetracycline, and others that your pharmacist or optometrist can tell you about).

"Ideally I would recommend lenses that block 100 percent of the UV rays below 390 nanometers in wavelength," says Dr. Sheedy. "Realistically, though, even some of the good materials might transmit 1 to 2 percent."

You can find this level of UV protection in both dark and clear lenses, both prescription and nonprescription. But the new excitement is over the recent Food and Drug Administration (FDA) approval of UV-protecting contact lenses. "There's an advantage to these because you're filtering out UV all the time—even on cloudy days when you might not normally wear your sunglasses," says Dr. Cannon.

Eyewear for Active People

The growing number of people who keep fit by exercising outdoors in the sunshine are also candidates for UV protection. But sports enthusiasts, in particular, have many other reasons to look to special eyewear and the growing field of sports vision.

"We're seeing more and more use of sunglasses to protect people not only from UV but also from strain," says Craig Farnsworth, O.D., project director of the Olympic Training Center's vision-testing and performance lab in Colorado Springs.

"It's pretty hard to squint in the sun all day and yet have your body be relaxed enough to play well and concentrate through a whole set of tennis or a round of golf. So we're seeing more distortion-free sunglasses that are also UV protected."

Certain lens tints can help in other ways, too. Many skiers, for example, find that special yellow tints make it easier to read the terrain accurately when lighting conditions are "flat," such as late on a winter afternoon, when the sun is low.

Use these tips to judge the quality of nonprescription sunglasses:

- Check to see if your eyes are visible through them. If they are, the sunglasses aren't dark enough. The lenses should screen out 75 to 90 percent of light. (This test won't work with light-sensitive lenses, though, because they are nearly clear indoors.)
- Hold the glasses at arm's length and look through them at a straight line, such as the edge of a door. Slowly move the lens across that line. If the straight edge distorts, sways, curves, or moves, the lens is not optically acceptable.
- Check to be sure that the lens tint is not darker in one area than another (gradient tints excluded) and that one lens is not darker than the other.
- Check the frame, the hangtag, or the case for the level of UV protection. If the information's not there, call the manufacturer.

A note of caution to young people, though: "Dark sunglasses can be addicting," says Dr. Farnsworth. "The eyes become less comfortable with bright light, and the person keeps wanting a darker and darker pair. The younger they start, the greater the chance of this happening. So for kids, we recommend wearing hats with large visors."

Another boon to sports enthusiasts (and other eyeglass wearers) are the new polycarbonate materials. Back in the 1950s and 1960s, most lenses were made out of glass. Then plastic became more popular because it was lighter. But polycarbonate is even lighter than plastic. In addition, it's a better UV protector and provides much greater impact resistance. "For this reason it's the preferred lens for people who engage in athletics," says Dr. Sheedy. Polycarbonate frames are also preferred. If you regularly participate in sports, especially those that involve a projectile, such as racquetball or softball, ask your optometrist about sports frames. They're worth the investment.

Many people find that they need a special eyeglass prescription for sports, anyway. Take golfers, for example. "If they're taller than 5'3", their regular bifocals may interfere with seeing the ball," says Dr. Farnsworth. "They tend to lower their head to see over the bifocal, and when they do that, they restrict their shoulder movement or bump their head on their shoulder, so the ball appears to move."

The answer? Using either a single-vision lens for golf or wearing a golfer's bifocal. These special bifocals have a small segment of added power off to the side of one lens (the right one for right-handers and the left one for lefties). This area does not interfere with their play but can be used for reading a scorecard (by holding it up and looking off to the side to read).

If you're having a sports vision problem, talk to your optometrist. If glasses can't solve it, special exercises called vision therapy might. "The older tennis player, for example, tends to lose the ability to track the ball," says Dr. Farnsworth. "Tracking exercises can often take care of the problem without the need for special glasses."

What Works at Work

Eye wear can also be specially tailored to tasks you perform at work. Painters and carpenters often use special bifocals that have the near-vision segment at the top, for example. Off the job, it's back to regular glasses. If your job requires you to focus at one distance for a long period, your optometrist can provide you with glasses suited for the chore.

One of the most recent job-related assaults on the eyes is working at a computer screen, or video display terminal (VDT). People with minor vision deficits often see well enough in their day-to-day lives, but add the stress of VDT work and they begin to have trouble. Most can find relief with a mild lens prescription worn only on the job.

Or people who were already wearing glasses may find that they're not geared to the new VDT work. This is common with bifocal wearers. The near-distance segment of bifocals is usually designed to give a sharp focus at the normal reading distance of 16 inches. But VDTs are generally viewed at 21 inches. Innovative wide-band trifocals are a good solution. They have a wide segment for intermediate-distance vision that provides a full view of the screen, and smaller segments at top and bottom for distance and near vision.

While some companies are marketing lenses with special tints to make VDT work easier on the eyes, Dr. Sheedy feels these aren't very useful. "Any possible benefit of those is extremely small compared with solving the major problems: getting the proper prescription and the right 'ergonomics,' such as proper lighting and height of the screen," he says.

If you do a lot of night driving or have trouble with bright lights, the new antireflection coatings may be just what the doctor ordered. Applied to the front of the lens, they eliminate reflections from the surface of the glasses. Not only does this banish ghost images from oncoming headlights, but there's a cosmetic advantage, too—people see your beautiful peepers instead of reflections coming from your glasses.

The right glasses for the right job: The only way to get them is to thoroughly discuss your work with an eye care professional.

Contacts for Better Health

Some of the most amazing technological leaps are being made in the field of contact lenses:

- Disposable contact lenses are already on the market. The lenses are worn for a week or two, then discarded in favor of a fresh, clean pair. "The theory is that you've got a clean lens, so it's healthier for your eye," says Dr. Cannon. "They also eliminate the need for cleaning and disinfecting solutions, which compensates for some of the cost."
- Medicated contact lenses are currently in the experimental stage. Their mission: to treat infections that are hard to get rid of with regular eyedrops. The lenses store medication and release it slowly into the eye. "The concentration remains higher over a longer period of time, so it has a higher cure rate than eyedrops," says Dr. Cannon.
- "Bandage" lenses are sometimes used to protect the eyes

of people with corneal problems. "This clear contact lens helps keep the eye from becoming infected," explains Dr. Cannon. "It's larger and thinner than a normal contact lens and reduces the pain that the lid causes as it moves across the tender eye."

- Soft lenses for color-vision deficiency (color blindness) are currently awaiting approval by the FDA. "These red lenses help people with some types of color blindness to discriminate colors better," says Dr. Cannon. They've been available in glasses and hard contacts for some time, but because they're red, most people find them too unattractive to wear. The developers of the soft-contact version say it is less noticeable and more comfortable.

- Orthokeratology is a treatment that uses a series of contact lenses to reshape the eye and overcome nearsightedness (myopia). The goal is to improve vision to the point where lenses are unnecessary for extended periods of time. The main application is for people in occupations where unaided vision is preferable: pilots, lifeguards,

What Optometrists Can Do for You

Optometrists perform eye examinations (you should have one every year), diagnose vision disorders and eye disease, treat eye problems, and write prescriptions for lenses. (For the most part, it's opticians, not optometrists, who fill prescriptions and sell lenses, including the nonprescription kind.) If you have a serious eye malady or need eye surgery, they can refer you to an ophthalmologist. The American Optometric Association, with a membership of 19,000-plus practicing optometrists, promotes eye care health education for the public and works to improve the quality and availability of eye care.

and athletes, for example. The drawbacks are that it doesn't work for everyone and the results are not permanent. "You have to wear a retainer lens to maintain the benefit," says Dr. Cannon. "You either sleep with it on or wear it for some time during the day, so you're never completely free of lenses." Still, orthokeratology may be worthwhile for people who have an occupational need, and it is safer than the equivalent surgical procedure (radial keratotomy).

- Fluorocarbon lenses may very well be the healthiest contacts ever. They are hard but are more oxygen-permeable than the plastic lenses that have been used until now. "The fact that this new material lets more oxygen through allows the cornea to maintain a more healthy, normal condition behind the contact lens," says Dr. Cannon. These new lenses are available right now.

PART III:
UPDATE ON CANCER

Flash Reports

DETECTING TINY TUMORS

Radio-tagged antibodies are helping doctors find even tiny cancers these days. The antibodies are injected into the bloodstream. They collect in cancer cells, where they can then be detected by a probe that detects radioactive emissions. The probe gives off a high-pitched whistle when it's passed over a cancerous area.

"We use the technique during surgery," says cancer surgeon Edward Martin, Jr., M.D., of the Ohio State University College of Medicine, where it was developed. "It can detect tiny tumors, tell us how far along they are, and help us determine the boundaries of a cancerous area." The technique is now being used for breast, colorectal, pancreatic, and ovarian cancers.

HIGH-TECH MACHINE
ZAPS CANCER

If conventional radiation treatment for cancer is a shotgun, then the new proton accelerator is a high-powered rifle. Unlike conventional radiation equipment, which sends x-rays completely through the body, the proton accelerator can focus its beam in three dimensions. It can deliver minimal radiation as it enters the body, then zap the tumor with maximum strength—and stop there. Because healthy tissue gets little exposure, patients suffer fewer side effects.

Proton accelerators are not new—they were developed for physics research in the 1940s. But the first one designed specifically for medical use is now being tested and will eventually be installed at Loma Linda University, in California. In the past, scientists made their research accelerators available to selected cancer patients, treating tumors that could not be eliminated by conventional radiation and surgery. For tumors of the eye, the cure rate has been 95 percent. For certain tumors at the base of the brain and along the spine, it is 80 percent, according to James M. Slater, M.D., chairman of radiation sciences at Loma Linda. Scientists now hope to be able to treat a wide variety of cancers with the new machine. "This is an unusual opportunity in cancer therapy," says Dr. Slater.

FIGHTING BLADDER CANCER

Scientists have found a new use for Calmette-Guérin bacillus, the organism used worldwide in tuberculosis vaccine. In a study of 86 patients who underwent surgery for noninvasive bladder cancer, half received the bacillus as part of their treatment and half did not. It was both infused into the bladder and injected into the skin. After five years, only 3 of the bacillus patients had died, compared with 13 of those who got surgery alone. "It works and it's highly effective," says Harry W. Herr, M.D., associate attending surgeon at Memorial Sloan-Kettering Cancer Center. It seems to work by stimulating the immune system. Although it's still being investigated, the researchers hope that the bacillus will be available for this use in the near future.

IMPROVING ON BREAST SURGERY

The carbon dioxide (CO_2) laser is now being used to perform breast cancer surgery. Advantages: The laser seals small blood vessels, eliminating heavy bleeding and reducing postoperative drainage. It also delivers intense heat to the area, which lowers the infection rate to near zero. And it leaves the surrounding tissue intact. "As a result, there's less pain following surgery," says Vincent W. Ansanelli, Jr., M.D., breast surgical oncologist in Great Neck, New York. Patients usually leave the hospital in one to two days following major breast surgery.

Even more important, animal studies have shown a significant decrease in subsequent breast cancer when the laser is used. Although this hasn't been proved in humans yet, studies are planned.

CHAPTER 15

Newest Weapons in the War on Cancer

Researchers at Roswell Park Memorial Institute in Buffalo, New York, offer new hope for cancer patients.

Cancer has long been one of the most dreaded words in our language. To many of us it sounds more like a death sentence than a diagnosis. Yet the latest news about cancer is anything but frightening. In fact, today there is no reason to let fear get the best of us, delaying diagnosis and treatment. The advances in cancer prevention, detection, and treatment make the prognosis look brighter than ever.

Prevention campaigns that focus on known risk factors, such as smoking, excessive sun exposure, and low-fiber diets, are already lowering cancer risks. New methods of early detection and treatment are increasing survival rates, even for some persistent types of cancer. Innovative therapies promise to do away with some treatments that seem almost as bad as the disease. Finally, research on human genes is dispelling some of cancer's mystery, telling us who's at risk, why, and what we may be able to do about it.

Here, then, is the hopeful news we've been waiting for. Some of the techniques described here are available already at hospitals and treatment centers across the country. Others are still experimental but available to those willing to try a new drug or treatment under rigorous medical supervision before it receives Food and Drug Administration (FDA) approval for widespread use.

Treatment Triumphs for Women

M. Steven Piver, M.D., chief of gynecologic oncology at Roswell Park, has developed a treatment that hasn't failed once in 25 years among women with early-stage uterine cancer.

As many as 10 percent of women who undergo hysterectomy to treat uterine cancer subsequently develop cancer in the vagina. Fortunately, this depressing statistic can be reduced with Dr. Piver's simple postoperative treatment: A small cylinder containing radioactive pellets is placed in the vagina after surgery and removed 48 hours later. This was recently listed as the standard treatment by the Physician's Data Query (a computer list of current treatments), but it's still not known and used in some hospitals!

A new double-pronged attack has made impressive inroads in curing cervical cancer: One prong is radiation therapy, and the other is a drug called Hydrea (hydroxyurea), given in twice-weekly doses during radiation treatment and for about a month following it.

In a double-blind test, 94 percent of the hydroxyurea patients were alive five years after treatment, compared with 53 percent in the control group on radiation and a placebo (dummy pill). Hydrea is widely available, but because this is a relatively new therapy, some doctors don't know about it.

Simply bringing this information to the doctor's attention may help many women benefit from the most advanced treatments available.

A Vitamin Boosts a Colon Cancer Drug

A ground-breaking tactic that combines a cancer drug with a vitamin is now being tested to treat colon cancer. The drug is 5-fluorouracil (5-FU); the vitamin is leucovorin, a form of the B vitamin folate.

The drug has been used for about 30 years in treating colon cancer. It slows cancer growth by latching onto an enzyme needed for cell reproduction. By itself, 5-FU is moderately effective. Add leucovorin, and it's much more effective, since the vitamin helps the drug bind more strongly with the enzyme. In one study, patients with incurable colon cancer survived about six months longer when given 5-FU and leucovorin.

New Drug Delivery Systems

One of the most impressive new techniques has been developed to fight cancers in the abdominal cavity, where almost half of all cancers begin.

Researchers have been looking for ways to deliver higher concentrations of drugs directly to such cancer cells, both to increase tumor-killing efficiency and to minimize the shock to normal tissue. One experimental but promising solution is intraperitoneal chemotherapy.

The organs of the abdomen (stomach, liver, intestines) are encased in a balloonlike layer of tissue. Now doctors can fill the abdominal cavity with fluid containing chemotherapy drugs, leaving them in until they're absorbed by the body. As the drugs go to work on tumor cells, they also get into the liver, where cancer often spreads first. The fluid can be drained and replaced several times for more intensive therapy. Another advantage: Higher-than-usual concentrations of most drugs can be used because treatment is more localized than normal chemotherapy.

A new and still experimental aspect of this therapy is to start it right in the operating room—immediately after tumor removal surgery. "That way, you can destroy any free-floating cancer cells that might remain, as well as treat microscopic areas where the cancer may have spread," explains Susan G. Arbuck, M.D., a research clinician at Roswell Park.

Children may benefit especially from intra-arterial chemotherapy, another method of delivery that limits side effects. A cancer drug is injected directly into the artery feeding the tumor. This concentrates the drug's effectiveness, minimizing dosage so less of the drug circulates throughout the body, according to Martin L. Brecher, M.D., acting chief of pediatrics at Roswell Park.

This therapy has also helped save arms and legs. Osteogenic sarcoma, a bone tumor that primarily occurs during adolescence, doesn't respond well to radiation. Formerly, the treatment of choice wasn't much of a choice: amputation. Now intra-arterial chemotherapy may be used to shrink the tumor to the point where it can be removed without taking the rest of the limb with it. A prosthetic bone implant is manufactured to fill in the missing segments.

A Drug Helps Lasers Zap Tumors

Solid-tumor cancers may become easier to treat with the development of a new technique that combines a drug with a laser.

The drug, hematoporphyrin derivative (HpD), has two special properties: It's absorbed very well by tumors, and it causes a destructive chemical reaction inside cells when it's exposed to light, especially the concentrated light of a laser. HpD has one significant side effect: It makes skin extremely sensitive to sunlight for one to four months. For the patient, that means covering exposed areas when outside and keeping out of sunlight shining through windows.

Despite this drawback, HpD seems to be an extremely safe and effective way to kill tumors, according to the drug's developer, Thomas J. Dougherty, Ph.D., a cancer research scientist at Roswell Park. The patient receives an injection of the drug, and doctors wait two or three days for it to clear from the blood. The tumor, which retains a significant amount of the drug, is exposed to laser light, often delivered through a fiberoptic scope. Large tumors may take several treatments, or may be "debulked" surgically before this procedure.

The FDA has approved HpD for use against lung, bladder, and esophageal cancers in clinical trials. More preliminary trials are planned or in progress for other types of solid-tumor cancers. The prime challenge now is to find a dose low enough to minimize sun sensitivity yet high enough to be effective.

Antibody Factories

An innovative diagnostic method has been developed that uses antibodies to detect tumors while they are still tiny enough to escape detection by other means.

When you get sick, your immune system makes specific antibodies against the invading organism that caused that illness. If the same "bug" infects you again, the antibodies recognize it, bind to it, and trigger white blood cells to attack it. Monoclonal antibodies are laboratory-made antibodies that can recognize specific types of cancer cells. They're produced by injecting mice with human tumor cells. When the mice make antibodies, the antibody-producing cells are removed from their spleens. These cells are then genetically combined with an *immortal* cell line (cancer cells that keep reproducing indefinitely). The result is an antibody factory in a test tube.

The potential uses of monoclonal antibodies are staggering. They can be tagged with harmless radioactive particles and injected into the body to diagnose cancer. A scanning device called a gamma camera may be able to find clusters of the radioactive-tagged antibodies too small to be found by other means. There is some danger of the patient having an allergic reaction to the mouse proteins that make up the antibodies, but in practice, most people merely get an annoying case of hives that can easily be treated. Researchers predict that commercial diagnostic kits may be available to doctors within a year.

Much further off, but still promising, is the use of monoclonal antibodies to treat cancer. Powerful cancer-killing drugs and radioactive substances can be attached to monoclonal antibodies and transported directly to a tumor. Doctors at Roswell Park are just beginning to explore this type of therapy in humans.

Another natural substance found in the blood of lab mice, tumor necrosis factor (TNF), seems to act against tumors several ways. According to Enrico Mihich, M.D., director of the cancer drug center at Roswell Park, TNF can kill cancer cells; it can rally other natural killers to the attack; and it seems to increase the effect of the chemotherapy drug Adriamycin. Right now TNF is still in preliminary clinical trials to determine its effectiveness.

Genetic Research: Holy Grail

Perhaps the ultimate question in cancer research is "What went wrong?" A cell mutates and grows beyond control. Why? We have some clues, but no one really knows—yet. One of the handful of people anywhere close to an answer is Thomas B. Shows, Ph.D., director of the Department of Human Genetics and cochairperson of the committee responsible for the worldwide registry of human genes, headquartered at Roswell Park.

Dr. Shows and his colleagues are trying to complete a map of the human genome: charting the location and function of all genes on our 23 pairs of chromosomes. We know the function of over 1,500 human genes, but that's only about 2 percent of the map.

Of special interest are oncogenes—genes that influence the development of cancer. Besides familial polyposis, a genetically determined tendency to develop hundreds of little polyps inside the colon, researchers can now test for the abnormalities that cause retinoblastoma (a cancer of the eye), neuroblastoma (a cancer of nerve tissue), Wilms' tumor (a kidney tumor), and chronic myelocytic leukemia.

Most questions in genetic research have yet to be answered, but as the map is filled in, so too is our understanding of the ways that good genes go bad. Gene-splicing techniques on individual cells have made high-tech treatments, such as monoclonal antibodies, a reality. Genetic cures—replacing an abnormal gene with one that functions properly—are still a long way off, however. But some day, this ground-breaking research might make cancer a benign, easily treated condition.

CHAPTER 16
A Guide to America's Best Cancer Treatment Centers

Centers sponsored by the National Cancer Institute are tops. Here's where they are and how you can contact them.

There's a lot of good news in the so-called war on cancer: new drugs, promising treatments that boost the immune system, improved surgical techniques, and more effective combinations of tried-and-true therapies. But to take full advantage of the latest knowledge and technology, you should contact a cancer center on the front line of the battle. Fortunately, there are more of them than you'd think. And one may even be in your area.

To locate the best cancer clinics, some of America's most respected physicians were asked this question: "If you or a member of your family had cancer, where would you go for treatment?" The unanimous answer: the nearest cancer center sponsored by the National Cancer Institute (NCI).

Why this unanimity of opinion among professionals in the know? What makes the NCI-sponsored programs the best?

NCI centers pioneer new treatments. All NCI centers conduct basic research. They also have large treatment facilities. This close relationship between research and treatment encourages rapid development of new and better treatments. (Of the 33 antitumor drugs commercially available, 24 were developed at NCI centers.) Staff physicians can follow a new drug or technique through research and get it to their patients as soon as it's considered safe and effective. This test stage of any new treatment is known as a clinical trial.

For certain types of cancer, clinical trials may offer a better alternative to standard treatment. Technically, a clinical trial is still an experiment. But it's a very safe experiment conducted under strict ethical guidelines. "No patient in a clinical trial receives anything less than the best care currently available," says Jerome W. Yates, M.D., associate director for clinical affairs at Roswell Park Memorial Institute in Buffalo, New York. "The patient gets either the standard therapy or a new treatment that in extensive preliminary testing is shown to be at least as good." And in many cases, newer is better.

The NCI sets the standards for cancer treatment. The National Cancer Institute maintains an up-to-date computer list of the most effective current treatments for each type and stage of cancer. It's called PDQ. (Yes, it does retrieve data Pretty Darn Quick, but the initials really stand for Physician Data Query.) Twenty-one NCI physicians and an oncology nurse specialist meet monthly to review and update the PDQ information. Their recommendations are based on their own experience, a review of current medical reports, and the experience of several hundred health professionals from cancer clinics around the country. PDQ's standards are America's standards.

The physicians at NCI centers are among the best in their fields. The centers attract highly qualified people because they have the equipment and funding to support extensive research programs. But it's more than a few outstanding individuals who make these centers so good: It's the team approach.

Today, cancer treatment is multidisciplinary. That means there's usually a combination of specialists involved: medical, radiological, and surgical oncologists, oncology nurses, and more. NCI centers have top people in each specialty. These physicians interact constantly, sharing their expertise and opinions with each other.

NCI centers are equipped to perform the latest cancer diagnostic and treatment procedures. This includes CAT scanning and magnetic resonance imaging (MRI), as well as laser-based procedures like the flow cytometer, which can count and separate thousands of cells per minute. Special techniques, such as bone marrow transplants, can be performed in only relatively few medical centers around the country. You are more likely to find high-tech equipment and specialized procedures at an NCI center.

Patients benefit from the support of the large NCI network. As of this writing, there are 20 comprehensive cancer centers, 21 separate clinical cancer centers (which treat patients but do less laboratory research than comprehensive centers), 15 basic research centers, and several hundred smaller groups associated with the main NCI headquarters and research facility in Bethesda, Maryland. All of these centers share their projects and results. A clinical trial begun at one center may enroll and treat patients at several others. All centers contribute data to the PDQ. If you go to one center, you have the resources of all of them at your disposal. That's probably the biggest advantage of all.

Good Care Is Always Available

This is not to say you can't get good care outside of an NCI-supported hospital. You can, if you choose carefully. You may find an excellent oncologist at your community hospital, for example. Also, some large non-NCI hospitals and university medical centers run their own clinical trials that are Food and Drug Administration approved and peer reviewed. It's important to note, too, that certain cancer treatments are so standardized, virtually any qualified physician can administer them with consistently good results.

The trouble is, cancer research is advancing so quickly that the newer and better treatments are not necessarily available at every institution. What the NCI network offers you, first and foremost, is assurance that the treatment you get at any of its affiliated centers is the best that's available today. You don't have to look any further.

How to Tap Into the Network

Here's how to make the NCI network work for you:

1. Look over the following list of NCI centers. If one is located near you, consider going there. You don't necessarily need a doctor's referral. You can check yourself in for a primary exam or a second opinion. If you've been diagnosed elsewhere, bring copies of your medical records along with you (or ask your doctor to make them available to whomever you see). Going to an NCI center puts the entire network at your immediate disposal. Chances are, you won't need to travel very far. Though some centers may have special research interests or programs of note, usually any one of them can give you the best available treatment for any kind of cancer.

2. Check with your local hospital to see if it's part of the NCI's Community Clinical Oncology Program (CCOP). At last count, there were 52 CCOPs, with 253 participating hospitals across the country. Your physician might be a participant in CCOP, too. Any doctor or institution involved in this program automatically shares information with the NCI clinical and comprehensive centers. It's "the next best thing to being there."

3. If your local hospital isn't part of a CCOP, you can call the nearest NCI center or dial the NCI cancer hotline (1-800-4-CANCER) to find out if there's one in a neighboring community.

4. If there's no NCI-connected institution in your area, your physician can still tap into the network. In fact, if you're going to be treated outside the NCI system, ask your physician if the treatment he or she recommends coincides with the standard treatments set down by the NCI. You should also inquire whether you might qualify for an NCI clinical trial. Any doctor who has a MEDLARS (National Library of Medicine computer

search program) hookup can answer both questions by tapping directly into the PDQ information network. The cost is around $15. Or your doctor can call the regional NCI center for a consultation. For that, all he or she needs is a phone.

5. All you need is a phone, too. You can contact the NCI centers yourself. Or for information about any aspect of cancer or treatment, call the NCI's toll-free hotline: 1-800-4-CANCER. In Hawaii, residents of Oahu can make a local call to 524-1234. From the other islands, call that number collect. Spanish-speaking operators are available during the day for callers from California, Florida, Georgia, Illinois, area code 201 in New Jersey, New York, and Texas. Information available on the hotline includes: Physician Data Query listings of standard treatments; PDQ listings of clinical trials, with all relevant contact information; member lists of physicians and hospitals involved in Community Clinical Oncology Programs; lists of NCI-approved cancer treatment programs at non-NCI hospitals. Booklets that explain various types of cancer and treatment are available on request.

For readable, practical advice for all cancer patients, many of the clinical directors we spoke with recommend *Choices: Realistic Alternatives in Cancer Treatment*, by Marion Morra and Eve Potts.

And now, the list.

New England

Dana-Farber Cancer Institute
44 Binney Street
Boston, MA 02115
(617) 732-3290 for patient information

The institute pioneered and developed treatments for childhood leukemia. Three different types of bone marrow transplants are used.

Norris Cotton Cancer Center
Dartmouth-Hitchcock Medical Center
2 Maynard Street

Hanover, NH 03756
(603) 646-5527 for patient information and/or referrals

Especially promising: intraoperative radiation and hyperthermia for pancreas and colon cancer, a unique program for brain tumors combining radiation implants with hyperthermia delivered through microwave antennae.

Roger Williams Center for Cancer and Related Diseases
Brown University
825 Chalkstone Avenue
Providence, RI 02908
(401) 456-2581 for patient information

Especially promising: bone marrow transplants in brain tumor therapy; lung cancer treated with a combination of drugs, radiation, and surgery.

Vermont Regional Cancer Center
University of Vermont
1 South Prospect Street
Burlington, VT 05401
(802) 656-4414 for patient information

Especially promising: intra-abdominal drug delivery for ovarian cancer.

Yale Comprehensive Cancer Center
School of Medicine
333 Cedar Street
New Haven, CT 06510
(203) 785-4095 for patient information and/or referrals

The first anticancer drug—nitrogen mustard—was discovered at Yale in the 1930s. They still have a very strong new-drug development program. Especially promising: combination of drug mitomycin and radiation for head and neck cancer; development of several new treatments for mycosis fungoides, a skin cancer.

Middle Atlantic

Albert Einstein College of Medicine Cancer Research
  Center

Chanin Building, Room 330
1300 Morris Park Avenue
Bronx, NY 10461
(212) 920-4827 or (212) 920-4826 for patient information

Especially promising: program for leukemia and lymphomas, including bone marrow transplants.

Columbia University Comprehensive Cancer Center
College of Physicians and Surgeons
701 West 168th Street
New York, NY 100322
(212) 305-6730 for patient referrals

This is one of the largest centers in the United States for brain tumor research and treatment. It offers ambulatory oncology care, a walk-in facility for continuous cancer treatment.

Fox Chase Cancer Center
7701 Burholme Avenue
Philadelphia, PA 19111
(215) 728-2570 for patient information

Especially promising: treatment of lymphomas, Hodgkin's disease, ovarian cancer with combination chemotherapy; comprehensive surgical management of pancreatic cancer.

Howard University Cancer Center
2041 Georgia Avenue NW
Washington, DC 20060
(202) 865-1406 or (202) 865-1408 for patient information
   and/or referrals

Extremely good cure rate and cosmetic results in head and neck cancers using combinations of drugs, radiation, and surgery; testing of same regimen on advanced cervical cancer.

The Johns Hopkins Oncology Center
600 North Wolfe Street
Baltimore, MD 21205
(301) 955-8964 for consultation information,

(301) 955-8979 for inpatient referral,
(301) 955-8964 for outpatient referral

(This is a national referral center for bone marrow transplantation and research. It has strong departments in childhood cancer and brain cancer.)

Memorial Sloan-Kettering Cancer Center
1275 York Avenue
New York, NY 10021
1-800-525-2225 for patient information, also
    (212) 794-7175 or (212) 794-7278 (8:00 A.M. to 5:00 P.M.
    Monday to Friday)

This is one of the original three models for the NCI comprehensive cancer centers and the largest private cancer clinic in the world. It has over 500 clinical trials ongoing at any one time.

Mount Sinai School of Medicine
Derald H. Ruttenberg Cancer Center
Fifth Avenue at 100th Street
New York, NY 10029
(212) 241-6361 for patient information

New York University Medical Center
Rita and Stanley H. Kaplan Cancer Center
550 First Avenue
New York, NY 10016
(212) 340-7227 for patient referrals

Especially promising: immune system boosters for brain tumors and ovarian cancer, an experimental "vaccination" process for melanoma (a particularly deadly skin cancer).

Pittsburgh Cancer Institute
220 Meyran Avenue
Pittsburgh, PA 15213
1-800-537-4063 for patient information

Innovative clinical trials, including a variety of immune system boosters, drugs, and a "vaccination" process for melanoma and renal cell cancers; intra-abdominal interleukin-2 (an immune booster) for ovarian cancer.

Roswell Park Memorial Institute
Elm and Carlton Street
Buffalo, NY 14263
(716) 845-2300 for patient information

This is one of the original three models for the NCI centers. The developer of a light-sensitive drug and laser treatment for certain tumors is at Roswell Park. Especially promising: an intravaginal radiation cylinder after surgery for early-stage uterine cancer; intraabdominal drug therapy for ovarian, colon, and stomach cancers.

University of Pennsylvania Cancer Center
7 Silverstein Pavilion (4283)
3400 Spruce Street
Philadelphia, PA 19104
(215) 662-6364 for patient referrals

Large treatment programs for breast cancer, melanoma, gastrointestinal, and colon cancers.

University of Rochester Cancer Center
601 Elmwood Avenue
Box 704
Rochester, NY 14642
(716) 275-4911 for patient information

This center was designed by the director, who planned everything for maximum comfort and privacy. It has its own library and art collection. Emphasis is on family participation, counseling, and a positive mental attitude.

Vincent T. Lombardi Cancer Research Center
Georgetown University Medical Center
3800 Reservoir Road NW
Washington, DC 20007
(202) 687-2110 for patient information

Most of the NCI's breast cancer research team moved here
with the center's new director.

South

The Cancer Center of Wake Forest University at the
   Bowman Gray School of Medicine
300 South Hawthorne Road
Winston-Salem, NC 27103
(919) 748-4464 for patient information

Especially promising: internationally recognized research
in antileukemia drugs, research in hyperthermia and drug
interactions with radiation.

Duke Comprehensive Cancer Center
Box 3843, Duke Medical Center
Room 228
Jones Research Building
Research Drive
Durham, NC 27710
(919) 684-5613 for patient information

Especially promising: large bone marrow transplant program for patients on drug therapy, experiments with immune boosters and hyperthermia.

Medical College of Virginia
Massey Cancer Center
Virginia Commonwealth University
MCV Station, Box 37
Richmond, VA 23298
(804) 786-0449 for patient information

Especially promising: bone marrow transplants for leukemia, lymphomas, other adult cancers, childhood malig-
nancies, and brain tumors.

St. Jude Children's Research Hospital
332 North Lauderdale
Memphis, TN 38101
(901) 522-0300 for information

Specializing in virtually all childhood cancers, following long-term survivors into adulthood (but anyone over 18 not accepted for initial treatment). Patients are accepted by physician referral only.

University of Alabama Comprehensive Cancer Center
Wallace Tumor Institute
1824 Sixth Avenue S.
Birmingham, AL 35294
(205) 934-6614 for patient information

Especially promising: extremely active research program testing monoclonal antibodies (natural immune system boosters).

University of Kentucky Medical Center
Lucille Parker Markey Cancer Center
800 Rose Street
Lexington, KY 40536-0093
(606) 257-4500 for patient information

Especially promising: bone marrow transplant and immune boosters.

University of Miami Medical School
Sylvester Comprehensive Cancer Center
1475 Northwest 12th Avenue
P.O. Box 016960 (D8-4)
Miami, FL 33101
(305) 548-4800 for patient information

Especially promising: development of an artificial bladder to replace some ostomies (ileostomy), testing of many new multiple-drug therapies.

University of North Carolina at Chapel Hill
Lineberger Cancer Research Center
School of Medicine
Chapel Hill, NC 27599
(919) 966-3036 for patient information

Areas of special interest: lymphomas, leukemia, and ovarian cancer.

University of Texas
M. D. Anderson Cancer Center
1515 Holcombe Boulevard
Houston, TX 77030
(713) 792-2121 for information

This is one of the original three models for the NCI centers and the nation's largest outpatient chemotherapy center. It has the largest interferon (an immune booster) research program in the world and the world's largest research program studying metastasis (how cancer spreads). Especially promising: voice-saving surgeries, lifelike prostheses for head and neck cancer surgery patients, limb salvage techniques for bone cancers. Patients are accepted by physician referral only.

University of Virginia Medical Center
Cancer Center
Box 334
Charlottesville, VA 22908
(804) 924-2562 for patient information

The center has a gamma knife, a device that uses focused radiation to perform brain surgery without cutting open the skull. Especially promising: hyperthermia with drugs and radiation for melanoma; a new, cosmetically acceptable treatment for a rare nasal cancer (ENB, or esphesioneuroblastoma); strong bone marrow transplant program.

Midwest

Case Western Reserve University
Ireland Cancer Center
2074 Abington Road
Cleveland, OH 44106
(216) 844-3980 for patient information

Especially promising: bone marrow transplant and high-dose chemotherapy for colon cancer; immune-boosting tumor cell "vaccination" for colon cancer; other immune boosters for cancers of kidney, ovary, pancreas, and skin.

Illinois Cancer Council Comprehensive Cancer Center
36 South Wabash Avenue
Suite 700
Chicago, IL 60603
(312) 346-9813 for patient information

No treatment is done at this address. The consortium refers patients to local member hospitals.

Mayo Comprehensive Cancer Center
Mayo Clinic, East 12
200 First Street SW
Rochester, MN 55905
(507) 284-3413 for patient information

Within a year, Mayo will have a gamma knife, a device that uses focused radiation to perform brain surgery without cutting open the skull. Mayo has the country's largest radiation therapy center.

The Ohio State University Comprehensive Cancer Center
410 West 12th Avenue, Suite 302
Columbus, OH 43210
(614) 292-5022 for patient information

Especially promising: bone marrow transplants; long-term survival rates with a new surgical approach to cancer that has spread to the liver, nicknamed the Swiss cheese effect.

University of Chicago Cancer Research Center
5841 South Maryland Avenue
Box 444
Chicago, IL 60637
outside Illinois, 1-800-482-6917 for patient information;
   in Illinois, 1-800-572-3692

The center is among the best in the country for Hodgkin's disease, non-Hodgkin's lymphoma, and leukemia. It has a world-renowned research program in secondary leukemia (which may occur after treatment for other cancers). It has treated over 500 patients with hairy cell leukemia, an extremely rare form of the disease.

University of Michigan Cancer Center
101 Simpson Drive, Box 0752
Ann Arbor, MI 48109
(313) 936-2516 for patient information

Especially promising: bone marrow transplant for small-cell lung cancer (and others); intra-arterial chemotherapy with radiation for liver and brain cancer; immune-boosting tumor cell "vaccination" coupled with other biological substances for cancers of skin, kidney, and esophagus.

University of Wisconsin Clinical Cancer Center
600 Highland Avenue
Madison, WI 53792
(608) 263-8600 for patient referrals

Especially promising: new techniques in brain surgery; bone marrow transplants; hyperthermia; and dramatic limb-saving operations for bone tumors, including at least one case of pelvis reconstruction.

Wayne State University School of Medicine
Meyer L. Prentis Comprehensive Cancer Center
P.O. Box 02188
Detroit, MI 48201
(313) 745-4400 or (313) 993-0335 for patient care referrals

This center is studying chemical carcinogens and the ways cancer spreads through the body. It has a strong breast cancer program and extensive experience with cancer in blacks. Especially promising: immune boosters for kidney cancer and melanoma, bone marrow transplant.

Mountain and Southwest

University of Arizona College of Medicine
Arizona Cancer Center
1501 North Campbell Avenue
Tucson, AZ 85724
(602) 626-6372 for patient information

Areas of special interest: multiple myeloma (a bone cancer), lymphoma (cancer of the lymph nodes), breast cancer, melanoma; promising work with immune boosters.

University of Colorado Health Sciences Center
University of Colorado Cancer Center
4200 East Ninth Avenue, Box B171
Denver, CO 80262
(303) 270-8801 for patient information

This center has a unique, large second-opinion clinic where patients can come in with slides and x-rays. It has extensive experience treating melanoma. Especially promising: trials with newest biologic agents, unique trial of high-dose radio-labeled antibodies in advanced breast cancer.

University of Utah Medical Center
Utah Regional Cancer Center
50 North Medical Drive
Salt Lake City, UT 84132
1-801-581-8793 for patient information

Especially promising: a unique *precision radiation therapy* for postmastectomy treatment, radiation implants for obstetric/gynecologic and head and neck cancers.

Pacific

City of Hope Cancer Research Centers
Beckman Research Institute
1450 East Duarte Road
Duarte, CA 91010
(818) 357-9711, extension 3292, for patient information

Especially promising: large bone marrow transplant program for leukemia and lymphoma; breast-preserving surgery and program for breast reconstruction shortly after surgery. Patients are accepted for evaluation regardless of ability to pay (unique). Aggressive treatment is their byword.

Fred Hutchinson Cancer Research Center
1124 Columbia Street
Seattle, WA 98104
(206) 467-4302 for patient information

Unlike other NCI centers, treatment concentrates only on bone marrow transplants for leukemia, lymphoma, aplastic anemia, certain deadly bone cancers, and pancreatic cancer spread to the bone.

UCLA Medical Center
Jonsson Cancer Center
Louis Factor Health Sciences Building
10833 LeConte Avenue
Los Angeles, CA 90024
(213) 825-1532 or (213) 825-5268 for patient information

Especially promising: immune system boosters, active hairy cell leukemia investigation.

University of California, San Diego, Medical Center
UCSD Cancer Center
225 Dickinson Street, H811-K
San Diego, CA 92103
(619) 543-6178 for patient information

UCSD has the largest lung cancer laser surgery program in the United States. It specializes in urinary tract cancers (prostate, bladder), brain and central nervous system cancers, and pancreatic cancer surgery. Especially promising: intra-abdominal drug therapy for ovarian cancer.

University of Southern California
Kenneth Norris, Jr., Comprehensive Cancer Center
P.O. Box 33804
1441 Eastlake Avenue
Los Angeles, CA 90033-0804
(213) CANCER-0; in Southern California, toll-free 1-800-5-CANCER for patient information

Especially promising: "vaccination" with immune boosters for melanoma; chemotherapy as an adjunct to surgery in bladder cancer.

Final Facts

Don't let fear of the disease or ignorance of the facts keep you from getting the best cancer care available.

You've got time. We've all heard that early diagnosis of cancer saves lives. An early-stage cancer—one that hasn't started to spread throughout the body—is easier to treat. But no cancer spreads so rapidly that you don't have some time to check your treatment options. In fact, you may jeopardize the success of your treatment if you don't take the time to think things through. "The initial treatment is the most important one," says John E. Ultmann, M.D., director of the University of Chicago Cancer Research Center. "It's your best chance for a successful outcome."

That's especially true for the up-and-coming cures: If you've had initial treatment, you won't be eligible for some clinical trials. That's because a new treatment must be tested on its own merits—without being hampered by previous therapies. So get as much information as you can (and discuss it with your doctor) before deciding on treatment.

You may not have to travel. There are 42 major NCI-supported treatment centers. They all offer the best standard treatments and clinical trials for any type of cancer. Even if a particular clinical trial is based at another center, you may be able to get the new treatment through a branch near you.

If you are not near one of these NCI centers, you may be able to get into an NCI clinical trial at a local hospital. That's especially true if your local hospital is part of the NCI's Community Clinical Oncology Program. Each CCOP includes several community hospitals and, in many cases, private oncology practices. They provide up-to-date treatments on the community level.

The only times you must travel a great distance are (1) if your treatment includes the use of specialized equipment only available at a few centers; (2) if a clinical trial requires you to be at a specific center; and (3) if you live in Alaska, where there are no NCI centers of any kind.

You can afford the best. In cancer treatment, *best* doesn't mean significantly more expensive. The first thing you should do is check with your insurance company to see what is covered. If you are concerned that an experimental clinical trial may not be covered—don't worry. The experimental treatment in an NCI-sponsored clinical trial is free. (Charges for routine hospitalization and physician care, however, are not.) And if you qualify for treatment under one of the specialized investigations at the National Cancer Institute's own main research center in Bethesda, Maryland, all your costs incurred during hospitalization are picked up by the NCI. Travel is covered, and lodging and food may be partially reimbursed.

You can be cured. There has been considerable progress in treating several types of cancer. Testicular cancer, for example, used to be considered one of the deadliest. It's extremely curable today. That turnaround happened because a few ordinary people volunteered to undergo a clinical trial—and refused to give up hope.

Above all, the war on cancer is fought with information. Arm yourself with the best advice available. It will make a difference.

CHAPTER 17

Update on
Skin Cancer

Knowing the warning signs of the near-epidemic cancer can save your life. When detected and treated early, it can almost always be cured.

Her lover first noticed the small, dime-sized black patch just below Elizabeth Williams's left breast. "It was a mole that had turned almost black," Williams recalls. "I wasn't really alarmed until I went to a dermatologist and saw the look on her face. Then I got scared."

The dermatologist diagnosed the tiny patch as malignant melanoma, the most deadly form of skin cancer. In 1984, the year Williams was diagnosed, 18,000 North Americans also learned they had skin cancer. Just three years later, the American Cancer Society estimated that 44 percent more—or 26,000—had malignant melanoma. For more than 7,800, the disease was fatal.

Skin Cancer Epidemic

Malignant melanoma is increasing in North America at near-epidemic rates. Scientists aren't sure why. Since the 1930s, the number of new malignant melanomas diagnosed each year has climbed more than 700 percent. Mortality from the disease has climbed as well. Today, more than 25 percent of those who develop malignant melanoma die from it.

Experts say that less-threatening skin cancers are also on the rise. According to the American Cancer Society, in 1987 about 500,000 North Americans developed basal or squamous cell carcinomas.

That's the bad news. The good news is that, if detected

and treated early, skin cancer can almost always be cured. Even better news is that by taking simple precautions, you can significantly reduce your risk of contracting skin cancer, and you can learn to detect it quickly if it does occur.

Cancer Types

The most common and least dangerous form of skin cancer is basal cell carcinoma. Although it cannot spread to other parts of the body (metastasize), it can extend below the skin's surface to the bone and cause considerable damage.

Squamous cell carcinoma, the next most common and dangerous type, differs from basal cell cancer in that it can spread and damage other parts of the body.

Malignant melanoma, the most dangerous skin cancer, begins when pigment-producing cells, melanocytes, begin to mutate and reproduce rapidly. The altered melanocytes continue to produce melanin, which accounts for the cancer's appearing in shades of brown, red, black, and navy blue. If untreated, melanoma can invade the lymph nodes and other vital organs, making it more difficult to treat later on.

All types of skin cancers occur most frequently in fair-skinned people who live in sunny climates, work indoors, and spend much of their recreational time outdoors. Those with family histories of skin cancer are also at increased risk.

People with lots of moles, particularly those irregular in shape, have a higher risk of developing malignant melanoma. Some researchers think that melanoma is triggered by acute, short-term doses of ultraviolet radiation, such as when people who work indoors spend two-week vacations getting suntanned. One group of researchers from the National Cancer Institute found that children exposed to just one blistering sunburn were twice as likely to develop melanoma later in life.

Elizabeth Williams fit the high-risk skin cancer profile perfectly. Born in Britain, Elizabeth spent her childhood summers in sunny Spain. "When the sun came out, everyone in my family would rip their clothes off and do this strange ritual of sunbathing," she says. "We'd compare to see who had the darkest tan."

Blond, blue-eyed, fair-skinned Williams says she got sunburned and peeled at least once a year as a child. "I think British people soak up the sun because we see the sun so rarely in Britain," she says. "When the sun comes out, we go nuts about it."

In 1982, Williams moved to Southern California. For the next two years she spent at least part of every day at the beach. She also spent a lot of time outdoors bicycling, hiking, and running. Shortly before she learned she had malignant melanoma, Elizabeth had a squamous cell lesion removed from her face.

Sun Connection

The time Elizabeth Williams spent in the sun probably had a lot to do with both her squamous cell cancer and her malignant melanoma. Experts say that overexposure to the sun's ultraviolet rays causes virtually all basal and squamous cell cancers. While the causes of malignant melanoma appear more complex, sun exposure plays an important role. "There's no question," says John Epstein, M.D., clinical professor of dermatology at the University of California, San Francisco, "sunlight accelerates melanoma."

Most malignant melanomas occur on the back and shoulders. In women, they also occur on the calves, areas not always exposed to the sun. Scientists note that melanomas occur more frequently in people who take summer and winter vacations.

Other researchers link increasing rates of melanoma to the depletion of the Earth's protective ozone layer. Ozone in the stratosphere, 12 to 21 miles above the Earth, shields us from some of the sun's ultraviolet rays. Emissions of chlorofluorocarbons, chemicals found in aerosol sprays, refrigerators, and air conditioners, are thought to be thinning the ozone layer, increasing the solar ultraviolet radiation. Recently, scientists found a hole the size of the United States in the ozone shield over Antarctica. Medwin Mintzis, M.D., assistant professor of dermatology at the New

York University School of Medicine, warns that every 1 percent increase in ultraviolet radiation reaching the Earth's surface could mean 2 percent more skin cancers. Increased exposure to sunlight does not fully explain the rise in malignant melanoma rates. "There seem to be other issues contributing to melanoma increases," says Dr. Epstein, "such as increased chemical carcinogens in the form of air pollutants and industrial emissions." Dietary polyunsaturated fat—recommended to help prevent heart disease—may also contribute to the rise in skin cancers. Scientists in Australia who compared 100 melanoma sufferers with 100 controls found that the cancer patients had higher levels of polyunsaturates in their fat tissues.

Self-Care

Whatever the causes, skin cancer rates are expected to climb during the next several years. Experts say that shielding your skin from the sun's ultraviolet radiation is the single most important protection against skin cancer.

"You don't have to avoid the sun completely," says Faye Arundell, M.D., clinical professor of dermatology at Stanford Medical School and board member of the American Academy of Dermatology. "You can do everything under the sun you want—except get a suntan."

Dermatologists say that it's especially important to protect children from the sun. Skin cancer rarely occurs in childhood, but recently it has become more common among people in their twenties and thirties. Most people receive 80 percent of their lifetime sun exposure before age 20. Reducing children's exposure to ultraviolet rays can significantly decrease the risk of developing adult skin cancer.

Parents should keep infants under six months covered or in the shade. If infant sunblock is needed, Dr. Arundell recommends zinc oxide. "It's a wonderful sun blocker," she says. "It even comes in colors now."

The American Academy of Dermatology suggests that older children be taught the "ABCs" of good skin care:

- A—Avoid midday sun (11:00 A.M. to 3:00 P.M. in the summer, 10:00 A.M. to 2:00 P.M. in the winter) when the highest amount of cancer-causing ultraviolet radiation reaches the Earth.

- B—Block the sun with a sunscreen with a sun protection factor (SPF) of at least 15. Apply the sunscreen liberally, and reapply every 60 to 90 minutes, more frequently after swimming or exercise.
- C—Cover up with hats and long-sleeved clothing.

The Best Protection: Sunscreens

Although sunscreens with sun protection factors up to 33 are now available, dermatologists say that SPF-15 sunscreens give most people all the sun protection they need.

A sunscreen's SPF refers to the amount of time it takes to get a mild sunburn while wearing it. For example, a fair-skinned person wearing no sunscreen at noon might develop a mild burn with 30 minutes of sun exposure. With an SPF-15 sunscreen, she'd have to spend 15 times as long—or 7½ hours—in the sun to get the same mild burn.

While you can pay more for the so-called super sunscreens with extra-high SPFs, most people don't spend enough time in the sun to warrant using sunscreens higher than SPF-15. "After SPF-15, you don't get much more protection," says University of California, San Francisco dermatologist John Epstein, M.D. "If you're extremely sun sensitive, however, a higher SPF may work for you."

Dermatologists also discount the idea of "building up" a tan to protect the skin from sudden, unavoidable sun exposure. "The deepest tan," says Stanford University's Faye Arundell, M.D., "has a sun protection factor of only 2 or 3." The best advice, she says, is to "wear sunscreen with sufficient SPF for your skin."

Adults should follow the ABCs of skin care, too. Dr. Arundell recommends that people with irregular, possibly precancerous moles be examined every three to six months by a dermatologist. Those with a family history should visit a dermatologist once a year. And everyone should do skin self-exams monthly.

Avoiding tanning booths is another item in the list of precautions. The booths use mostly the nonburning ultraviolet-A (UVA) radiation, which is less dangerous than ultraviolet-B (UVB) radiation, which causes sunburn. However, "UVA exacerbates the sunburn effect of UVB," says Dr. Epstein. "In animal studies, UVA radiation has also increased the cancer-causing effects of UVB rays." Spending 30 minutes in a tanning booth exposes you to as much UVA radiation as you'd get in half a day outdoors.

Dr. Arundell says people have misconceptions about suntans. "Society thinks people with suntans are healthy, but tanning damages the skin," she says. She hopes North Americans follow the example of "Doonesbury" character Zonker Harris and give up suntanning. "Suntanning is a social habit that can be changed," she says. "It took 30 years to convince people that smoking is unhealthy. It may take a while, but we hope to make suntanning socially unacceptable."

Since doctors removed her malignant melanoma three years ago, Elizabeth Williams has been careful to protect her skin from the sun. Though she's had no cancer recurrence, it's always in the back of her mind, and she frequently looks for skin changes. "I've changed my whole life around," says Williams. "I moved from southern to northern California to avoid the constant sunlight." At first, she tried to avoid the sun completely. Though she's resumed her outdoor activities, she always wears a high-SPF sunscreen. "I'm incredibly careful," she says, "Malignant melanoma is scary stuff."

CHAPTER 18

Zap Prostate Cancer

Tiny radioactive "seeds" release radiation into a targeted area.

One out of every three men over the age of 50 will get it—cancer of the prostate, a life-threatening condition that, until just recently, has required surgery, chemotherapy, or externally administered radiation therapy as a cure. But thanks to the ingenuity of the Theragenics Corporation of Atlanta, Georgia, men now have a very promising new option. The new therapy requires only local anesthesia, can be done on a outpatient basis in about 45 minutes, and—best of all—preserves sexual potency and fertility in most cases. The treatment is even relatively inexpensive. At about $8,000, it's roughly half the price of surgery and the same price as radiation therapy administered externally.

So what's the catch?

We couldn't find one, unless you want to consider the importance of early detection a catch. The therapy is not effective against tumors that have reached advanced stages. But then, the success rates of even the traditional treatments for prostate cancer drop off dramatically in cases where the disease is advanced, points out Harold P. McDonald, Jr., M.D., who's been successfully employing the new therapy in his clinic in Georgia for over a year now. "The procedure stands to have a major impact on this very widespread problem, but men are going to have to take it on themselves to be examined for the disease."

Radiation from the Inside Out

How exactly does the new treatment work?

"Using ultrasound as a positioning guide, we inject tiny capsules containing radioactive palladium into the prostate," Dr. McDonald explains. "For approximately 17 days, the capsules release the major dose of radiation, then gradually become inert. The 17-day period, however, is usually enough to effectively destroy the tumor in most cases. Once killed, the tumor then shrinks, the dead tissue gradually is absorbed by the body."

Not only is sexual potency usually left intact following treatment, but patients also tend to experience fewer problems with urinary incontinence and rectal or bladder irritation than with other types of therapy, Dr. McDonald says.

Success rates for the procedure?

"Although the technology has only been available for a year, we expect success rates to be as good as with the other available therapies," Dr. McDonald responds.

As for the implanted seeds—20 or more of which may be needed, depending on the size of the tumor—"they remain in the prostate," Dr. McDonald says. "They're harmless once they've become inert."

And what about the potential danger of having radiation emanating from within, even if it is for only 17 days?

"That's the beauty of the palladium capsules," he says. "They emit their radioactivity for only a very short distance, several centimeters at most. This assures that radioactivity remains localized to the cancerous tissue being treated."

Early Detection Is a Must

As with any treatment for prostate cancer, early detection is crucial, Dr. McDonald emphasizes. He recommends a complete examination of the prostate at age 40, with checkups every year after that. "This initial exam should include an ultrasound exam and a blood test in addition to the standard digital exam," Dr. McDonald says. "Early detection is vitally important with prostate cancer because if a man waits until he experiences symptoms (for example, frequent urination, back pain, or difficulty in stopping or starting urination), it's usually too late for a cure by any method."

The implant procedure is so new that only a few centers in the United States are currently set up to do it. Dr.

McDonald's Georgia Prostate Center is one. For more information on the therapy, including its availability in other parts of the country, contact Dr. McDonald at the Georgia Prostate Center, 2550 Windy Hill Road, Suite 215, Marietta, GA 30067 (404) 951-8466.

Flash Reports

BEAT
THE DIGITALIS BLUES

If you're a heart patient on digitalis and you've got the blues, you may be able to beat them with a simple change in your medication.

In a new study, researchers at Mount Sinai School of Medicine in New York found that 11 of 18 heart patients taking digitalis were depressed. The people had trouble sleeping and eating and had a reduced sex drive. Other patients taking different heart drugs were far less likely to experience depression.

"It used to be thought that people who took digitalis were depressed because they were so sick," says William Slater, M.D., the study's main researcher. He advises depressed patients on digitalis to ask their doctor about this possible reaction. The physician may consider stopping the drug for a time or switching to a different drug to see if the symptoms leave.

SUBLIMINAL MESSAGES
SPEED RECOVERY

Even when they're anesthetized, patients sometimes hear what's going on during an operation. Though they usually can't recall what they heard (unless they're hypnotized), the words still apparently have impact.

English doctors recently found that this phenomenon could be used to their patients' advantage. They studied a group of 39 women, all undergoing hysterectomies. During the operation, about half the women listened to blank tapes. The others heard tapes with positive messages, such as "You will not feel sick; you will not have any pain"; "The operation seems to be going well and the patient is fine"; and "How quickly you recover from your operation depends upon you—the more you relax, the more comfortable you will be." Neither doctors nor patients knew in advance which tape a patient would hear.

The results? Women who heard the positive-message tapes spent less time in the hospital, had fewer days of postoperative fever, and were less likely to have problems with gas, diarrhea, or constipation than women who'd heard the blank tapes. They were rated as having a better-than-normal recovery by nurses who didn't know which tapes the patients heard.

The researchers speculate that the tapes may have reduced anxiety by obscuring operating-room conversation and noise. That could mean that less anesthetic was needed, reducing the risks of complications. Or, they say, the state of awareness sometimes experienced during anesthesia may make people more open to suggestion, just as they'd be while under hypnosis.

ASPIRIN REVERSES STROKE DEMENTIA

The first treatment for stroke dementia, the loss of mental or cognitive ability after a stroke, may already be in your medicine chest. In a study of 70 patients at the Veterans Administration Medical Center in Houston, one aspirin tablet (325 milligrams) a day reversed dementia to the point that the patients no longer needed supervision. Test scores measuring cognitive ability showed a 17 percent improvement the first year, followed by a 21 percent improvement the second year, and 20 percent the third. By comparison, patients who received no aspirin showed no improvement, and some got worse.

The results were so dramatic that the researchers halted the trial after 15 months for ethical reasons, according to John Stirling Meyer, M.D., professor of neurology at Baylor College of Medicine.

Note: Aspirin should not be taken by stroke patients without a doctor's advice.

CHAPTER 19

New Migraine Tamers

Headache research is giving credence to remedies from the age-old to the newfangled.

True or false: People get migraines because they're perfectionistic, keep their anger bottled up inside, and don't make time for themselves.

Answer: Many migraineurs (migraine sufferers) do fit this classic image, but many are also relaxed and easygoing. "All kinds of people can get migraines," says R. Michael Gallagher, D.O., a Chicago-based headache specialist. Although stress and psychological factors definitely play a role, research is showing that migraine is an illness involving the brain's pain network. And the brain chemical serotonin—a substance that may help to moderate pain—is now science's number one suspect.

Another myth bites the dust. And so it goes, as the new boom in migraine research and treatment continues. Powerful new drugs are being developed. Headache clinics and inpatient hospital treatment programs are springing up across the country. Headache doctors are treating people more successfully, thanks to their increased understanding of migraine.

Here are six new ideas to come out of all this activity—and why they may help you overcome "the pain in the brain."

Monitor Medication

For many migraineurs, painkillers spell relief. But experts have recently discovered that the overuse of these drugs can also cause migraine through a kind of rebound effect. This knowledge has given migraine sufferers and doctors a powerful new antiheadache weapon.

All painkilling drugs are on the potential overuse list: aspirin, ibuprofen, acetaminophen, and other over-the-counter pain medications; prescription painkillers; and the ergotamine drugs, such as Cafergot, which are specifically prescribed for migraines. Migraineurs often live in fear of the next attack. So it's understandable that painkillers could become a fact of life. "Some patients start with two pain pills a day and end up taking many more than that, just to feel okay," says Joel R. Saper, M.D., a Michigan-based headache specialist. That buildup may happen in two ways. Mistake number one: dosing a mild headache with medication designed for a severe one. Mistake number two: using painkillers too frequently or as preventive medicine, hoping to ward off a headache that hasn't even arrived.

Why the bad rebound effects from generally helpful drugs? "The evidence so far suggests that chronic use of pain medication somehow impairs the transmission of serotonin," says Ninan Mathew, M.D., a headache specialist based in Houston.

The key word is *chronic*. These medications may all be very effective against head pain if taken occasionally according to your doctor's orders. "Two days a week seems to be the cutoff point," says Dr. Saper. More often than that and you're asking for trouble. Best bet: Take painkillers two days in a row (if necessary), so your body has five medication-free days in between. If you need more medication than this, you should probably consider a preventive therapy.

Here are the clues that indicate that your migraines may be related to overuse of painkillers:

- The frequency of pain is increasing, and pain occurs more than one or two days out of the week.
- You're using painkillers more frequently.
- You usually get a headache within several hours to a day after your last dose of painkillers.
- You're experiencing a dependable rhythm of medication, pain, medication.

To get off this rebound roller coaster, you have to break the painkiller habit, which is far from easy, because it means undergoing serious withdrawal pain. Sometimes hospitalization is necessary. The next step: an individually tailored treatment plan, which often includes preventive drugs. These drugs don't cause a rebound effect. Among the options: beta-blockers, calcium channel blockers, and tricyclic antidepressants.

In many cases, painkillers may safely reenter the picture. "Not everybody has to be on preventive medicine, and about half of migraineurs can come off their preventive drugs eventually," says Dr. Saper. But it may take weeks or months before the body's pain mechanism is back on track. In the meantime, preventive drugs can serve as a bridge to a saner, safer control of migraines.

Consider Feverfew

The aromatic herb feverfew is a folk "cure" (actually a preventive) for migraine. Recently, a group of English researchers at the University of Nottingham put it to the test, studying its effect on 60 migraineurs. Every day for four months, half the headache sufferers received a feverfew capsule and half received an inactive capsule. Then the groups switched treatments for another four months. While taking feverfew, the participants got an average of 24 percent fewer migraines, with no reported side effects. Vomiting was also reduced. So was the severity of the attacks.

The scientists speculate that feverfew may affect serotonin—the chemical most specialists believe is centrally involved in migraines. But more research is needed to confirm or rule out feverfew as useful therapy. If you want to try feverfew, do so under your doctor's supervision.

Relax to the Music

Biofeedback is a form of behavior training that allows people to consciously control certain body processes usually regarded as beyond conscious manipulation. It's a well-established preventive for headache. And, according to some experts, it's especially useful for migraine patients who can't take medication. Now preliminary evidence at least suggests the possibility that listening to music may be another behavioral therapy for preventing migraines.

In a study at California State University in Fresno, 30 migraine sufferers were divided into three treatment groups. The first group used biofeedback. (In this case, the subjects were taught to warm their hands by changing their thoughts. Hand warming helps divert blood flow from the head, which presumably is what helps lessen the likelihood of migraine.) The second group listened to music—either classical or "easy listening." The third group was a control group that received no treatment at all.

Both the biofeedback and music groups also learned progressive muscle relaxation, gave themselves positive suggestions, and practiced visualization techniques in which they imagined that their headaches had a physical form that could somehow be destroyed or counteracted. Both groups trained in these techniques (plus either biofeedback or music listening) for five weeks with two 40-minute sessions per week, for a total of ten sessions.

One year later, the results were surprising. The music-listening group had fewer migraines than either the biofeedback group or the control group. And the migraines they did have tended to be slightly shorter and less severe than those in the other two groups.

Why the difference? The effect was probably not related to music itself, says Janet E. Lapp, Ph.D., who ran the study. It turns out that the music group simply practiced more often. When they listened to albums at home or heard tunes throughout the day, the music served as a cue to relax and practice their visualization. These constant "refreshers" helped them improve their skills over the course of the year.

Experts are quick to point out that this small study doesn't prove that music therapy is a better bet than biofeedback. More studies are needed to compare the benefits of biofeedback and music for migraine sufferers. Meanwhile, Dr. Lapp says, if you want, you can try the music treatment yourself. Throughout the day, whenever you hear music, associate it with peaceful thoughts and a pain-free head. In addition, set aside 15 minutes every day as "your time." Turn on some music you find relaxing. Sit in a comfortable chair or lie down. Relax every part of your body, from toes on up. Then let go of every troubling thought. Simply rest and listen. One caution, though: If your headaches don't improve, don't hesitate to consult a physician.

Catch On to Caffeine

Headache scientists now understand that caffeine has a good side and a bad side. On the good side (which a lot of migraineurs take full advantage of), there's the fact that a couple of strong cups of coffee (or glasses of caffeine-containing soft drinks) plus some over-the-counter pain medication may stop a migraine in its tracks. Caffeine tends to enhance the absorption of pain medication from the intestine. (That's why many painkillers contain caffeine.)

You have to consider this remedy an *occasional* option, though—to be used no more than twice a month. It simply won't work if you're a longtime heavy caffeine user. That's because once you've built up a tolerance, your body won't notice the jolt of caffeine.

Which brings us to the dark side of caffeine. Heavy, daily caffeine use (over 500 milligrams a day—about five cups of coffee) can create a painfully vicious cycle. That is, a migraineur who drinks lots of caffeine may get more frequent migraines, which may be relieved by more caffeine (at least until tolerance), and so on.

Scientists think there are two reasons for this roller coaster of pain. First, caffeine is a stimulant—that is, it stimulates certain brain cells to secrete chemicals that relieve pain. But constant stimulation of brain cells may cause them to get tired out and therefore reluctant to release the brain chemicals. And without the pain-soothing chemicals, your head continues to ache.

Second, there's caffeine's effect on blood vessels. Drink some regular coffee and your blood vessels constrict. Since migraine is associated with dilation of blood vessels, the presence of caffeine may tend to keep pain at bay. But several hours later, as caffeine leaves the body, blood vessels may dilate—setting the stage for a migraine. This effect is seen most often in heavy caffeine users. That may be why many migraineurs who rely on caffeine during the day wake up with a headache every morning.

So to deal effectively with the dual nature of caffeine, experts say, quit entirely (except for occasions when you try the caffeine remedy) or reduce your intake. Nobody knows what the safe limit of intake is for migraineurs, in part because people have different tolerances. But some migraine specialists recommend no more than one cup of coffee per day—about 85 to 150 milligrams. At this intake, you're likely to be able to avoid the treacherous cycles of pain and relief yet use the caffeine-painkiller cure about twice a month.

Smokers, Take Heed

Here and there, clinicians are beginning to suspect that cigarette smoking worsens migraines. Although no formal studies have been done, some doctors strongly advise their migraine patients to quit.

How could smoking incite a migraine? For one thing, smoking releases carbon monoxide. And whenever carbon monoxide shows up, people get headaches. Also, nicotine—another bad guy—gets into your system. It actually interferes with some of the drugs used to control migraines, such as beta-blockers and antidepressants. As a result, doctors often have to increase the dosages, which can lead to more side effects.

Look Out for MSG

About 20 percent of migraineurs can trigger a migraine by eating the wrong thing. Migraine experts have known for years that one of the substances that does this triggering is monosodium glutamate (MSG). And the most disturbing—and most useful—news for those few who react to MSG is that it's in things you would never suspect.

We now know that MSG (a natural substance) is added to hundreds of processed and "natural" foods. And all too often, it's a hidden ingredient.

The Food and Drug Administration (FDA) requires that MSG itself be listed on a food label. That part's easy—MSG-reacting migraineurs can just bring their reading glasses to the supermarket and read labels. Classified as a flavor enhancer, MSG is often added to soups, broths, sauces, gravies, spice blends, canned and frozen meats, poultry, and vegetables.

The problem comes when a given ingredient contains some MSG. In such cases, the FDA does not require the manufacturer to tell you so. For instance, the flavoring agent called hydrolyzed vegetable protein (often listed as HVP, and sometimes called protein hydrolysate or hydrolyzed plant protein) always contains MSG—and is sometimes up to 20 percent MSG. HVP is found in bouillon, dried soups, imitation bacon bits, croutons, frozen dinners, most seasoning salt, and canned tuna. (You can, however, wash most HVP out of the tuna.)

Even "natural flavors" can contain MSG. HVP is considered a natural flavor and may be listed as such. Kombu, a seaweed most often found in Japanese-style foods like miso or ramen soups (as an extract or powder), contains MSG. That's why an announcement of "all natural ingredients" on food packages is no guarantee that the product is MSG free.

Is there enough MSG in these foods to actually trigger a migraine in a sensitive individual? Research indicates that people differ widely with regard to their MSG sensitivity. To determine your own tolerance level, keep a diary and look for connections between your migraines and the intake of certain foods. "Most migraine sufferers who are sensitive to MSG will respond to it within 24 hours," says

George R. Schwartz, M.D., a physician based in Santa Fe and the author of *In Bad Taste: The MSG Syndrome.*
If you are sensitive to MSG, here's how to avoid it when you eat out:

- Call the restaurant first and inquire about the ingredients they use, especially hydrolyzed vegetable protein. Find out whether the foods include prepackaged mixes— they're likely to contain MSG. Soy sauce is 10 percent MSG.
- MSG is more easily absorbed on an empty stomach. So start your meal with an appetizer that is likely to be MSG free, such as fresh fruit or a plain roll.
- Steer clear of sauces and gravies.
- When ordering, just say "no MSG." Even if the chef uses seasoning salt (with MSG) instead, you may end up with a lower dose.
- When dining on a plane, order broiled fish or a low-salt meal, both of which are less likely than meat or chicken to contain added MSG. Check the ingredients in salad dressings carefully. Peanut snacks may contain MSG. So can the luncheon meats used in snack sandwiches ("natural flavoring" or "flavorings" on the package of cold cuts may mean MSG).

CHAPTER 20
All about Alzheimer's

For caregivers and others, a guide to understanding this complex disorder and meeting the needs of the patient.

Two-and-a-half million Americans suffer from Alzheimer's disease, a progressive brain disorder that destroys the mind and takes the lives of more than 100,000 Americans annually. The disease currently ranks as our number four killer, behind only heart disease, cancer, and stroke.
The Alzheimer's jokes you laugh at when you're under

30 aren't so funny when you're over 40 and caring for a parent or spouse or fearing for yourself. "Alzheimer's disease is a disorder with monumental impact," agrees University of South Florida professor of psychiatry Eric Pfeiffer, M.D. "Nearly 10 percent of persons over age 65 have Alzheimer's disease, another 10 percent of this age group are caregivers to patients with Alzheimer's disease, and many of the remaining 80 percent live in daily dread that they may be among the disease's next victims."

Worse yet, the Alzheimer's epidemic is expected to increase dramatically in years ahead as the size of the elderly population continues to grow. Incidence of the disease is expected to triple over the next 50 years. Alzheimer's usually strikes after the age of 65, but people in their fifties and even forties can also be afflicted. The disease takes anywhere from 2 to 20 years to cause death.

What Causes Alzheimer's?

Is it in the genes? If a family member has succumbed to Alzheimer's, are your own risks increased?

Only if the family member's disease struck early—at the age of about 40—are you at greater risk, research indicates. "Alzheimer's disease that has its onset at age 40 may present a 40 percent risk for family members," reports J. Thomas Hutton, M.D., Ph.D., director of the Texas Tech Alzheimer's Disease Center and chairman of the Texas Council on Alzheimer's Disease and Related Disorders. "In contrast, Alzheimer's disease beginning after the age of 80 brings about little or no increase for the family member as compared with the general population."

The autoimmune hypothesis. Perhaps most intriguing of all is evidence suggesting that the body's own immune system may cause Alzheimer's disease. Normally the brain is protected from autoimmune responses (instances where the body's immune system turns against itself, such as with rheumatoid arthritis), but some research suggests that this protection system may break down with age. Events such as concussions or strokes may hasten the breakdown of the protection system (known as the blood-brain barrier), as may alcoholism and high blood pressure. The result of a blood-brain barrier breakdown may be that antibodies enter the brain and react to brain proteins in ways that produce the neural plaques and tangles characteristic of the Alzheimer's condition. The autoimmune hypothesis, while plausible, remains to be proven, however, Dr. Hutton says.

Could it be a virus? And what about recent findings suggesting a virus may be responsible for Alzheimer's?

"The strongest evidence linking Alzheimer's disease to an unconventional 'slow' virus infection results from the discovery that other rare neurological diseases previously thought to be degenerative in nature have now been shown to be caused by transmissible viruslike agents," Dr. Hutton says.

Efforts to prove that Alzheimer's acts similarly have failed up till now. However, some very preliminary results of a study done at Yale again raise the possibility that Alzheimer's is caused by some unknown infectious agent that circulates in the blood. The researchers took blood samples from people with two close relatives suffering from Alzheimer's as well as from a person who had early signs of it. Then they injected the white blood cell portion of each blood sample into hamsters' brains. Within a year the hamsters had developed a degenerative brain disease. However, much more investigation is needed before it will be known if Alzheimer's is caused by a virus or bacteria. "What does seem clear is that persons exposed to Alzheimer's victims do not have an increased chance of developing the disease," Dr. Hutton says.

The Need for Compassion and Humor

While scientists are uncertain of the causes and at least 10 to 20 years away from a cure for the memory and thinking disorders caused by Alzheimer's, there are effective ways to manage the disease and control its progress.

"Alzheimer's appears to be a very complex disease," says Richard J. Ham, M.D., of the State University of New York Health Science Center at Syracuse. "It causes neural

How Bad Is It?
Try This Test

Eric Pfeiffer, M.D., professor of psychiatry and director of the Suncoast Gerontology Center at the University of South Florida Medical Center in Tampa, devised the following questionnaire to assist in evaluating dementia. It may help you determine if you should be seeking further medical attention for a relative. (Question 4A is to be asked only if the patient does not have a telephone.)

1. What is the date today?
2. What day of the week is it?
3. What is the name of this place? (That is, where are you?)
4. What is your telephone number?
4A. What is your street address?
5. How old are you?
6. When were you born?
7. Who is the president of the United States now?
8. Who was the president just before him?
9. What was your mother's maiden name?
10. Subtract 3 from 20 and keep subtracting 3 from each new number all the way down.

For patients with at least some high school education but not more than high school education, the following scoring applies. (Allow one more error if the patient has only a grade school education; allow one less error if the patient has had education beyond high school.)

0–2 errors: intact intellectual functioning
3–4 errors: mild intellectural impairment
5–7 errors: moderate intellectual impairment
8–10 errors: severe intellectual impairment

plaques and tangles in the brain's delicate network of nerve cells that are distinctly different from changes that occur in the brain as it ages naturally. As good as we've been at defining these changes, however, we're still largely in the dark as to why they occur. I wouldn't want to discourage people from remaining hopeful that some degree of prevention will evolve, but I would emphasize the importance of learning to cope with Alzheimer's *today.* Good management is effective in reducing the symptoms of the disease."

For example: Encouraging a patient to reminisce about those aspects of his past that he can remember helps maintain a sense of reality and preserves social skills, Dr. Ham says. And helping to reduce the effects of a patient's deficiencies rather than reacting with anger can help minimize the depression, self-reproach, and withdrawal so characteristic of the disease.

"Just because a patient has lost the ability to communicate does not mean he has lost the ability to understand and regret his condition," Dr. Ham says. "It's important for caretakers to realize this."

A sense of humor also can be valuable in helping to lighten the burdens imposed by Alzheimer's, Dr. Ham says. This doesn't mean trivializing a patient's condition, of course, but it does mean being able to laugh sometimes when you could just as easily cry.

The Importance of Safety and Comfort

Just as important as the emotional aspects of caring for the Alzheimer's patient, however, are the physical challenges of the job. Because the Alzheimer's sufferer often lacks sound judgment in addition to deterioration of routine physical skills, his environment needs to be tailored accordingly. The following tips for ensuring maximum safety and comfort for Alzheimer's sufferers come from *Caring for the Alzheimer Patient,* edited by Raye Lynne Dippel, Ph.D., and J. Thomas Hutton, M.D., Ph.D.

To be sure the patient does not injure himself or herself:

- Restrict or monitor use of matches and lighters.
- Remove temperature controls from the stove if the patient is unsafe in the kitchen.
- Reduce clutter in rooms, and on floors especially, to minimize the risk of falls.
- Have the patient wear an identification bracelet.
- Remove keys to cars when the patient is no longer capable of driving.
- Suggest the patient put his mattress on the floor, thus making restraints unnecessary.
- Make certain stairs and hallways are adequately lit.
- Consider installing exit alarms if wandering becomes a problem.

To help make it easier and more comfortable for the patient to deal with limitations:

- Identify the bathroom with a picture or sign.
- Encourage the patient to use the bathroom at frequent intervals to avoid accidents.
- Provide laxatives or stool softeners if constipation is a problem.
- Supply an automatic dialing service so the person doesn't have to remember phone numbers.
- Encourage daily exercise.
- Avoid issues that result in explosive confrontations.
- Remove mirrors; they intensify anxiety if a person no longer recognizes himself or herself.
- Encourage all skills the patient may retain.
- Allow the patient to eat in privacy if he or she develops unacceptable eating habits.

Other Causes of Dementia

Although 50 to 65 percent of age-related mental impairment is due to Alzheimer's, other conditions can compromise intellectual functioning or produce Alzheimer-like symptoms. They can also make existing Alzheimer's worse. The main ones your doctor should consider are:

- Medication effects
- Depression

An Update on THA, the One-Time Wonder Drug

You may have read in your local newspaper of an experimental drug known as THA (tetrahydroaminoacridine). Several years ago, doctors and families of Alzheimer's patients were excited when a researcher noted improvement in patients given oral doses of this drug. The excitement quieted somewhat when the experiment was criticized for being limited in size and degree of control, but THA nonetheless was considered worthy of further study by the Food and Drug Administration (FDA). The trials were halted in early 1988, however, when THA was found to be toxic to the livers of some participants. Smaller doses of the drug are now being tested under the auspices of the National Institutes of Health's National Institute on Aging, but preliminary results were not available at this writing.

Will THA turn out to be the cure millions have been waiting for? Probably not, even if its liver toxicity can be ironed out, most experts agree. The drug may reduce symptoms of Alzheimer's in some patients, but it does nothing to cure the disease, just as insulin does nothing to cure diabetes.

THA is not available in the United States. However, a doctor with an Alzheimer's patient can apply to the FDA for permission to have the drug shipped from countries where it is on the market. In cases of desperate, terminal illness, the FDA sometimes allows the purchase abroad of drugs that are not legal in this country. For more information, have your doctor contact the FDA.

- Hypothyroidism or hyperthyroidism
- Alcoholism
- Multi-infarct dementia (senility caused by strokes)

Other causes of dementia include

- Brain tumors
- Kidney failure
- Liver failure
- Electrolyte imbalance
- Hydrocephalus (water on the brain)
- Huntington's disease
- Late multiple sclerosis
- Late Parkinson's disease
- Posttraumatic brain injury
- Pernicious anemia
- Neurosyphilis
- Creutzfeldt-Jakob disease
- Chronic fungal or tuberculous meningitis
- Pick's disease
- AIDS

CHAPTER 21

Sure-to-Soothe Agents for Body and Brain

Deep breathing, progressive muscle relaxation, and walking are just a few of the proven healers.

It's 3:19 in the afternoon. Your flight leaves at 3:23. You're ten minutes away from the airport. Or you would be, if traffic were moving. It isn't. A big truck just turned over. The highway is covered with melons—and state police cruisers.

As they say in the funny papers, "ARRRGH!"

Stress strikes at inconvenient moments, usually when the best ways of defusing it are impossible to employ. You can't always back off for an hour to meditate or hop into a flotation tank. You've got to get on a plane, or make a speech, and a wave of tension hits. You need something now.

So consider one of the following on-the-spot tranquilizers. Some are natural substances, some are drugs, some are techniques to trick yourself into serenity. But they're all designed to control your internal response to a stressful situation—in 30 minutes or less—when you can't do anything about the situation itself.

They can manage this in two ways. They can attack the physical symptoms of stress (pounding heartbeat, rapid breathing, tensed muscles). Anything that diffuses these physical responses will feed back through the nervous system and calm you. Or they can biochemically short-circuit the brain's stress response, which is primarily how a prescription tranquilizer works. Or they can work on both body and brain.

The tranquilizers here are arranged roughly in those groups: body, brain, or both. And within those groups, they're ranked approximately by tranquilizing power, from mildest to strongest. This ranking lets you select your calming agent according to a well-established medical principle: Try the gentlest treatments first, stepping up cautiously to the more potent options if you get no relief. This approach helps you avoid tranquilizer overkill and minimizes possible side effects.

Note: If your anxiety or stress is ongoing or particularly intense, see your doctor. A tranquilizer may not be the answer.

The Body Calmers

The following techniques will help call a halt to tension and let your body relax.

Breath control: the six-three-six method. Stress makes you breathe as if you had just run a 50-yard dash. Slow down your breathing and you control the stress response, experts say. Slower breathing—the kind you use in breath control techniques—even has a feedback effect that gradually makes your heart stop pounding. And the overall sense of control you get from such methods psychologically reinforces the calming effect. Besides, they're fast and easy. You can do them anywhere. And they have no side effects.

Here's a good one, called the six-three-six method, suggested by James Hackett, codirector of the Chicago School of Massage Therapy: Inhale for a count of six (one-thousand-one, one-thousand-two, and so forth); hold that breath (gently) for a count of three; exhale for a count of six. Repeat as often as necessary.

While you're doing the six-three-six, close your mouth and breathe through your nose. This automatically slows your breathing, since you're using a smaller "intake valve." And learn to breathe from the diaphragm rather than the chest muscles. The diaphragm draws air deeper into the lungs, making each breath more efficient. Test yourself: Put one hand on your chest and the other on your stomach just above your navel. If the lower hand is the only one moving when you breathe, then you're breathing correctly.

Muscle relaxation: the quick release. One popular stress reliever is progressive relaxation, a 20-to-30-minute regimen of tensing and relaxing various muscle groups. A shorter version of this technique, called the *quick release*, was developed by Robert H. Phillips, Ph.D., director of the Center for Coping with Chronic Conditions, on Long Island, New York. It combines breath control and muscle relaxation in a few easy steps.

1. Sit or lie down, and close your eyes. If you must stand, lean against something.
2. Inhale, and hold that breath for about 6 seconds while tensing as many muscles as you can.
3. Exhale with a "whoosh" and let your body go limp. Breathe rhythmically for about 20 seconds.
4. Repeat steps two and three (twice). After the third release, relax for about a minute, concentrating on a peaceful scene or visualizing the word *calm*.

The beta-blockers. It's difficult to play Beethoven's Fifth Symphony when your hands look like they're ready to shake, rattle, and roll. So when faced with preperformance heebie-jeebies, some concert musicians turn to a class of prescription drugs commonly used to reduce high blood pressure: beta-blockers. Musicians say that these drugs can quiet their pounding heart without significantly reducing muscle control or concentration. In fact, some claim that their playing improves—and there are medical studies to back them up.

Beta-blockers literally block the action of certain hormones that are released during stress. The most immediate effect is a reduction in heart rate, which causes blood pressure to go down and apparently yields a greater sense of calm. It's not surprising then that physicians prescribe beta-blockers for stage fright.

But are these drugs really safe to use as impromptu calmer-downers? Experts say yes, but only if the drugs are used once in a while (one dose before a performance, for example), only in healthy people (the drugs can be especially dangerous for diabetics, asthmatics, and people with glaucoma or certain heart problems), and only under a doctor's supervision. People who take beta-blockers daily for blood pressure control have reported side effects, such as lethargy, cold hands and feet, dizziness, depression, sleep problems, sexual dysfunction, diarrhea, and nausea.

The Brain Soothers

The remedies listed here have a calming effect on the brain.

Valerian: the root that relaxes. Modern medicine scoffs at many herbal remedies, but at least one herb has a scientifically tested tranquilizing effect. It's valerian, also known as garden heliotrope (*Valeriana officinalis*). Alvin B. Segelman, Ph.D., a pharmacognosist (one who studies the medicinal uses of plants) at Rutgers University, calls it "one of the few herbal tranquilizers that are proven safe and effective."

Overall, the herb has a fairly mild tranquilizing impact, with very few known side effects. Its worst characteristic is probably its pungent odor.

The Food and Drug Administration allows it to be sold as a food additive, so the herb is available in capsules, tinctures, and tea bags in many health food and herbal stores. Prices and potency may vary.

The problem with valerian, though, is that its active ingredients (called valepotriates) can vary greatly in concentration from plant to plant, or even within the same plant at different times of the year, which means that capsules can also vary in potency.

Getting an effective dose is often a matter of trial and error, according to Varro Tyler, Ph.D., a Purdue University pharmacognosist. As a general rule, though, he recommends that you limit your occasional intake to two cups of valerian tea (made by steeping fresh, chopped pieces of root in hot water for 10 to 15 minutes) or two 475-milligram capsules. Valerian is a hardy plant, so you can grow it in the backyard.

L-tryptophan and carbohydrates. A few years ago, researchers suggested that an amino acid called L-tryptophan may be "nature's sleeping pill." Since then studies have confirmed that tryptophan does indeed help insomniacs get to sleep faster. But can tryptophan work as a tranquilizer for those who want to stay awake?

"Yes," says nutrition researcher Judith J. Wurtman, Ph.D., from the Massachusetts Institute of Technology. "And the way to put tryptophan to work is to eat carbohydrates."

Here's why: When carbohydrates are digested, the pancreas releases insulin. In addition to regulating blood sugar, insulin decreases the bloodstream concentration of amino acids—except for tryptophan. Higher tryptophan levels then reach the brain, and the brain uses them to manufacture a chemical called serotonin.

"Serotonin is the calming chemical," says Dr. Wurtman. "When the brain is using it, feelings of stress and tension are eased."

Because digestion isn't an instantaneous process, there's a slight delay before you feel calmer. Dr. Wurtman says that some people feel better within 5 minutes after a carbohydrate snack. Most people feel calmer within 20 or 30 minutes. A small number of people feel little or no calming effect.

But we eat carbohydrates all the time. Why aren't we

calm and collected all the time? Because the fat and protein that we eat with them can interfere with the tranquilizing effect. Even the slightest amount of protein eaten with carbohydrates can prevent usable quantities of tryptophan from entering the brain. And fat can slow the digestion of carbohydrates, gearing down the whole tryptophan chain reaction.

The answer is to eat low-protein, carbohydrate between-meal snacks—foods like rice cakes, dry cereal, and air-popped popcorn. (Don't eat them with a glass of milk, though.) Most people need only 1 to 1;1/2 ounces of pure carbohydrates to produce a tranquilizing effect.

Alcohol. Most of us have had firsthand experience with alcohol's tranquilizing effects. On occasion, some of us may forget where tranquilization ends and barroom floor begins. From a more scientific point of view, alcohol tranquilizes because it's a powerful depressant that acts directly on the brain and because it's a mild muscle relaxer.

And for many healthy people (not those with a tendency to overdo it or to drive afterward), a drink or two can be an effective and relatively safe tranquilizer. So say a number of experts. But they also caution that a mild tranquilizing effect should be the goal. Beyond that, you risk intoxication, with all its accompanying social and health penalties. Besides, if you're under so much stress that just a little tranquilizing power won't do, you may need more than alcohol or any other tranquilizer can give. When your judgment is clouded by this much stress, it may be hard to stop at two drinks.

Two additional warnings: Alcohol in excess or in combination with certain drugs (especially prescription tranquilizers) can be lethal. And in chronic alcoholics, drinking can actually increase anxiety.

Brain-and-Body Relaxers

And now for some measures that can do double duty in the battle against stress.

The ten-minute walk. Can a little thing like a short, brisk walk have an immediate tranquilizing effect?

Apparently so, according to psychologist Robert Thayer,

Ph.D., of California State University, Long Beach. Dr. Thayer has performed several studies on the mood-altering effects of brisk ten-minute walks. His subjects reported a decrease in tension for up to one hour after walking. There was even a noticeable effect after walks only two or three minutes long! Yet the participants weren't sedated by the walks—in fact, they reported a boost in energy. Good news for those who want to calm down but not conk out.

How does the walking tranquilizer work? Surprisingly enough, the release of muscle tension seems to play only a small role. Endocrinologist Edward Colt, M.D., assistant professor at Columbia University in New York City, says that a chemical reaction in the brain produces the primary tranquilizer. Natural morphinelike substances called endorphins, which are released during exercise, account for much of the tranquilizing. Other brain chemicals are probably involved as well.

Perhaps there are also some psychological tranquilizers at work here. A brisk walk may give you the sense of stepping away from your problems. Or perhaps the mental solitude allows you to concentrate without distractions.

A big plus: There are virtually no side effects—unless you walk through the wrong neighborhood.

Hot baths. You've seen the commercial: "Calgon, take me away!" Hot baths have a tranquilizing effect, with or without the sponsor's product. In fact, according to Richard S. Gubner, M.D., medical director of Safety Harbor Spa and Fitness Center in Safety Harbor, Florida, "Hot baths are the oldest form of tranquilizer known." The tranquilizing effects are so powerful and so immediate that, until supplanted by drugs, hot baths were used to quiet violent patients in mental hospitals.

Hot baths are generally thought to work by relaxing the muscles. A recent study from Loughborough University in England, however, suggests that part of the effect may be caused by heating of the brain. The investigators say that hot baths that caused a 2°C rise in body temperature (about 1°F) later caused an increase in the deeper stages of sleep. Now researchers are investigating the effectiveness of hair-dryer hoods to heat the brain directly. (Maybe that's the secret appeal of the beauty parlor: tranquillity!)

Dr. Gubner says that if you have time to enjoy a hot bath, your bathwater should be about 100° to 102°F, and you should soak for no more than 15 minutes. *Do not* take a hot bath or shower immediately after a strenuous workout—give yourself time to cool down. And if you're taking vasodilating drugs for high blood pressure, consult your doctor before hopping into the tub. In either case, you could faint or experience heart problems. For most people, though, a hot bath is soothing and safe.

Prescription tranquilizers. The most widely used prescription tranquilizers in the nation belong to the chemical family that includes Valium and Librium: the benzodiazepine compounds. This family is the largest-selling drug group in the world. Many critics say these calming agents are overused.

Prescription tranquilizers do have a bad reputation, thanks in part to fiction like *Valley of the Dolls* and facts from the lives of a number of celebrities. That reputation is partly justified. Most of the older drugs (barbiturates, meprobamate) are addictive, and there's a danger of overdose with them.

The benzodiazepines, introduced in the mid-1960s, were an improvement. They are less addictive and less dangerous than earlier tranquilizers. They're central nervous system depressants and muscle relaxants—they relieve the mental and physical aspects of stress. Under most circumstances, they take effect within 30 minutes. Valium and Librium remain effective for about eight hours, but small amounts of these drugs can stay in the body for days. Newer benzodiazepines work up to six hours but are rapidly eliminated after that, preventing dangerous buildups.

Still, there are dangers: The most common side effects in occasional use include drowsiness, impaired coordination, dizziness, digestive problems, and headaches. Driving can be a problem: Studies have shown significant impairment on a moderate dose (15 milligrams per day) of Valium, for example. And any prescription tranquilizer can be lethal when combined with booze. "These drugs compound the effect of alcohol," says psychopharmacology specialist Jacob J. Katzow, M.D., an associate clinical professor of psychiatry at George Washington University and director of the Washington Clinic for Mood Disorders. "It's a case of one plus one equaling three."

And, of course, the potential for addiction is ever present in long-term use. Some people can become dependent on Valium in a few weeks. Withdrawal symptoms from these drugs can be serious, especially if they are stopped cold. To prevent this, the dosage is usually tapered off over a few weeks.

Despite their possible drawbacks, however, prescription tranquilizers are generally strong, effective, and relatively safe on a short-term basis. But they should be used only under a doctor's supervision.

The newest Valium-type tranquilizer, Xanax (alprazolam), seems to be the safest. Dr. Katzow calls Xanax a "significant improvement" because it doesn't make patients as drowsy as Valium does. Xanax recently overtook Valium as the largest-selling prescription drug in this country.

There are also some nonbenzodiazepine drugs that deserve mention, if only because you may have heard of them. Quaaludes (methaqualone) are no longer manufactured in this country. They were widely abused. Barbiturates (which date back to the beginning of the century) and meprobamates (marketed as Equanil and Miltown) are sometimes used in patients who don't respond to Valium-type compounds. And a new drug, BuSpar (buspirone hydrochloride), seems to be an extremely safe alternative to Valium. Unfortunately, BuSpar doesn't seem to have an effect until it's been taken regularly for a week or more. Perhaps a faster-working compound will be isolated in the future.

A Tranquilizing Footnote

One final tip: "The healthiest form of stress reduction is humor." So says Paul Jay Fink, M.D., chairman of psychiatry at Albert Einstein Medical Center and president of the American Psychiatric Association. It's easier to deal with stress if you don't take yourself too seriously and don't view every problem as a life-or-death situation. We often laugh at stressful situations—when they happen to somebody else. If you can train yourself to see the humor in your own situation, you'll distance yourself from the problem and feel you have more control.

So if you can, laugh. And if you can't, then reread this chapter.

CHAPTER 22

Getting Out From Under the Threat of Panic Attacks

Working with a trained therapist is usually the answer.

Waiting in line at the supermarket, Brenda is seized by panic. For no reason—out of the blue. A feeling of unreality and impending doom floods her mind. Her heart rate jumps sky-high. She feels like someone's holding a pillow over her face. She knows if she doesn't get out of there, she's going to die or go crazy. Leaving the cart in the line, she walks quickly to her car and drives home. In the safety of her living room, she calls her family doctor, certain that she's had a heart attack.

What she's really had is a classic first panic attack: a sudden onslaught of anxiety and fear for no apparent reason. Without effective treatment—and there's plenty available—Brenda's likely to have other attacks. And suffer emotionally and socially under the threat.

Some experts say panic disorder (when severe panic attacks recur frequently and disrupt your life) is one of the most common psychiatric disorders in the country, affecting maybe 5 percent of Americans. The typical sufferer is a woman in her twenties whose first attack occurred in her late teens, says Christopher McCullough,

Ph.D., director of the San Francisco Anxiety and Phobia Recovery Center. The attacks last from 5 minutes to an hour, averaging 15 to 20 minutes, with minor attacks much shorter. The average panic disorder sufferer gets them two to four times a week, but people have been known to get as many as several a day and as few as one a year.

Sufferers is an apt description of people who have true panic attacks. They get depressed because they can't lead normal lives. To relieve their anxiety and depression, some start taking drugs or alcohol and end up abusing them. They often have insomnia and then can't stay awake in the daytime.

But you've got to meet certain criteria to qualify as a bona fide panic "attackee." First, at least 4 of the 12 recognized symptoms have to be present: breathing difficulty, pounding heart, dizziness, tingling fingers and feet, chest pain or tightness, a smothering sensation, faintness, sweating, trembling and shaking, hot or cold flashes, a sense of unreality, and the ultimate whopper, a fear of dying.

Another prerequisite is that at least four of the symptoms must occur suddenly, "within 10 minutes," says David Sheehan, M.D., director of research and professor of psychiatry at the University of South Florida School of Medicine.

And the prime criterion, many experts say, is that the symptoms must occur without apparent cause. People who get panic attacks, for example, are often highly sensitive to caffeine. "But if you drink 20 cups of espresso, you're going to have a panic attack, no matter what," says Alexander Bystritsky, M.D., director of the Anxiety Disorders Program and assistant clinical professor of psychiatry at the University of California, Los Angeles. That's why, some say, a genuine panic attack has to occur out of the blue, with no stress in sight. You may panic on your first parachute jump, or when you're mugged, but who wouldn't? That's not a panic attack. That's pure common sense.

Looking for the Cause

Nobody really knows what causes panic attacks, but there are several competing theories.

The biological cause. Panic attacks often seem to be passed down from parent to child. It's possible that a person has a genetic predisposition for panic, and stress triggers it.

Another bit of evidence for a biological connection: Panic attacks are three times more common in women than men. "Another clue is that panic attacks in women are much less common after menopause," says Dr. Sheehan. "It's possible there's a gene involved inherited by both women and men, but for some reason women are more sensitive to it than men." Dr. Sheehan also notes that panic sufferers' resting heart and breathing rates are higher than normal, though they may not know it.

Then there's lactate and caffeine. An infusion of an amount of lactate (a normal biochemical by-product of exercise) equal to that produced in intense exercise can cause an attack in a sufferer but not in a normal person, Dr. Sheehan says. And people who get panic attacks need much less caffeine than nonsufferers to precipitate an attack.

The psychological cause. "We feel the roots go back to childhood insecurity," Dr. McCullough says. After 15 years of treating panic disorder exclusively, he says, "I see the same personality traits over and over again." There's been an actual or imagined separation or rejection from the parents, or maybe the parents were overprotective. Often they were alcoholics and gave confusing, on-and-off signals to their children. "From that very fundamental insecurity, the child develops a superstructure of strength and independence in order to survive. It serves her very well, but in early adulthood under heavy stress, she has a panic attack and is reduced back to this frightened child. It wrecks her self-image of independence."

Psychologists don't reject the biological theory altogether. They say some people may be more sensitive to biological factors because they're anxious.

The catastrophic misinterpretation cause. Proponents say some people misinterpret normal signals of anxiety, transforming them into a catastrophe. In fact, panic attackees, before having their first panic attack, are often able to tolerate more stress than normal, unaware they're under stress. So says Fred Wright, Ed.D., director of education for the University of Pennsylvania Hospital's Center for Cognitive Therapy. "In the mind of a person having a panic attack, rapid heartbeat equals heart attack, light-headedness equals brain tumor or stroke," Dr. Wright says.

So panic disorder sufferers often get every type of medical test offered, from electrocardiograms to electroencephalograms to CAT scans. "Being told that nothing is wrong with them doesn't help at all," Dr. Wright says. "Often they figure, 'That doctor doesn't know what he's talking about. I'm getting another opinion.' And third opinions and fourth opinions."

It's a classic description of hypochondria. And that's why psychiatrists like Dr. Sheehan challenge the misinterpretation theory. "Panic attack sufferers are accurately reporting their symptoms," he says. "I don't think they're misinterpreting at all. I think physicians are misinterpreting. They can't grasp the intensity and devastation of the symptoms. It's not hypochondria. It's a mismatch between the patient's and doctor's perceptions. To the patient, it is out of the blue. Sure, there's a snowballing effect. But it happens in any physiological symptom. Once the person realizes what's happening to his body, it becomes more extreme."

Dr. Wright says, "We might be lumping several disorders together under the same name. Someday we might get to the point where we can discriminate between different types of panic—one that clearly has origins that are genetic, or biological, or emotional, or the result of faulty learning."

From Panic to Phobia

Whatever the theory, the standard stresses—divorce, separation, a death in the family, moving, difficulty at work—are often known to precede a person's first panic attack, even though the patient might not link them to her attack.

This first panic attack is usually not recognized for what it really is. By the time the victim has exhausted all medical possibilities, he or she has usually had several more attacks. And these ensuing panic attacks are usually triggered—through simple association—by a place or event where he or she had a previous attack: a shopping mall, a bridge, an elevator, a cocktail party, driving a car, even in bed in the middle of the night. So the events and places become fearsome.

And this sequence of events is how two-thirds of panic attacks grow up to be phobias. "Almost all phobias begin with a panic attack or an anxiety attack of some sort," Dr. McCullough says.

Now when Brenda even thinks about a supermarket, she gets a little jittery and worries about having another attack there. So she figures she can avoid another attack by avoiding the supermarket. "This is how agoraphobia [literally, fear of the marketplace] begins," Dr. McCullough says. Avoiding the supermarket might work temporarily for Brenda, but since she hasn't worked on her real problem—whatever is really causing her panic attacks—she might get her next attack while driving. So she avoids driving. Then she worries she might get one in a restaurant, so she stops eating out. "Pretty soon you start avoiding everything to the point where you don't go out at all," Dr. McCullough says. If she keeps up this way, Brenda may eventually be afraid to come out of her bedroom. She will have become what Dr. McCullough calls "a successful phobic."

Treating Fear Itself

Divergent theories lead to divergent treatments. That's why it's essential, says psychotherapist Jerilyn Ross, president of the Phobia Society of America, "to be sure your doctor is open to many different ways of treating you. Many psychiatrists have begun to realize that medication is more effective with therapy for many people. And psychologists also realize that patients with severe panic attacks fare better when medication is used in conjunction with therapy."

Each person is unique, and the therapy has to be custom tailored. But in general, each method alone can help cut the number and intensity of attacks and can be even more effective in combination with the others. With help, you can banish these attacks altogether. And there are even ways you can abort an attack before it really has a grip on you.

Cognitive therapy. Dr. Wright and his colleagues at the University of Pennsylvania are pleased with their results using cognitive therapy (a nondrug, behavioral approach) to correct anxiety misinterpretation. Still under study, this treatment focuses on getting panic disorder sufferers to change their original way of thinking about and dealing with the sensations of anxiety. "What better way than to have them reexperience the panic and then show them that they have some control over it?" says Dr. Wright. "The primary goal is getting the person to experience the panic and see that nothing bad happens to them, without letting them go to what we call a safety zone, such as the emergency room or their house."

Cognitive therapy was developed for depression therapy by Aaron Beck, M.D., in the 1960s. It's now also being used for many psychiatric problems, including substance abuse, marital discord, and eating disorders. Dr. Wright's cognitive therapy approach is a several-step process.

"First, we educate the person about anxiety," Dr. Wright says. "Many people aren't sure what anxiety is all about. We show them that their physical symptoms are actually part of a survival mechanism—the fight-or-flight response."

The second step is to induce an attack in the doctor's office. (One way to induce is to use hyperventilation.) "We can't rely on recall of what someone thinks during an attack," Dr. Wright says. "So we have to re-create the experience." The therapist asks the person, "What's going through your mind right now?" The attackee may reply, "I'm going to die! I'm going insane! I have a brain tumor!"

On hearing the panicked replies, the therapist helps the person realize that the symptoms are due to normal anxiety instead of impending death. The therapist might say, "Yes, your heart is beating faster and you're breathing faster, but those are merely the physical symptoms of anxiety."

Later, the therapist induces another attack and shows the person how to slow her breathing down by listening to a tape of a normal breathing rate. When she slows her respiration to a resting rate of 8 to 12 in-and-out breaths per minute, the person notices that the sensations of panic dissipate. "If you were truly having a heart attack or stroke, controlled breathing wouldn't stop it," Dr. Wright says. "But if you're creating the symptoms and escalating them through hyperventilation, controlled breathing will stop them. Hyperventilation or hypoventilation—when you're breathing in gasps and holding your breath—occurs in 70 percent of panic attacks."

After all of the above steps are mastered, the person is then instructed to bring on a panic attack in the safety of her own home, or even in a place she associates with panic attacks—like Brenda's supermarket. "She then uses controlled breathing to help reduce the symptoms of the attack," Dr. Wright says.

At this stage, there's an even greater emphasis on objectivity. "We teach them to be more objective in the early stages of the sensations of panic," Dr. Wright says. "When they get up in the morning and have a cup of coffee and their heart starts beating faster, they tell themselves, 'I just drank some coffee, so of course my heart's beating faster. It's going to go away.'"

The last stage is to try to figure out what might have triggered the initial panic attack. "If the person is under continual stress, she's going to continue to have body sensations of normal anxiety," Dr. Wright says. "If she can find out what's causing the stress, she might be able to do something about it. But even if she can't, she can learn to cope and get on with her life."

By the end of cognitive therapy, Dr. Wright says, the panic attack sufferer has worked on all three parts of the disorder: the attack itself, worrying about having another one, and developing phobias. "The eloquent solution is when you've cured all three parts," he says.

Some people with panic disorder may be able to use cognitive therapy by themselves or with a spouse or friend, Dr. Wright says. But because of the need for education about panic and reassurance that there is no physical disorder, "The majority probably need help."

Psychotherapy. Dr. McCullough and other psychotherapists believe you have to go deeper to find a complete recovery. "There are all kinds of relaxation tapes and ways

to breathe, and they're an important part of treatment,"
he says. "But unless you deal with the underlying anxiety,
they're just Band-Aids."

Many people have been in deep psychoanalysis for years
with no improvement in their panic disorder. Dr. McCullough and other psychologists, however, practice what he
calls "short-term psychotherapy" that lasts a few weeks to
a year.

"It's literally a matter of 'reparenting,'" he says. "We
find specific ways to meet those unmet childhood needs
that stemmed from very early (15 to 22 months of age)
rejection or mixed signals from the parents." For example,
in desensitization therapy (where the person is gradually
exposed to things he thinks give him panic attacks), "I may
take a person with panic disorder and agoraphobia on a
field trip to a shopping center," Dr. McCullough says. "I
sit there in a coffee shop and she goes wandering off
like a child would, and when she becomes anxious and
terrified, she comes back and touches base with me. I give
her reassurance, which she didn't get when she was two
years old, and I nudge her to go back out. That's exactly
what a healthy parent would do."

He combines this minitherapy with cognitive therapy
and assertiveness training. "I don't think insight in itself
helps anybody," he says. "Some say if you have the insight, the behavior will take care of itself. Others say forget
the insight, just change the behavior. I think the combination produces a more authentic cure. When it comes to
assertion, we want the person to ask herself, 'How can I
take some risks in my world to be myself?' "

Medical therapy. A patient at Dr. Bystritsky's clinic will
get treatment corresponding to the severity of his panic
attacks. People with a mild disorder learn standard relaxation and breathing techniques—visualizing places or situations that make them feel calm, and controlling breathing
so they don't hyperventilate. Those with moderate panic
disorder can benefit from cognitive therapy, which focuses
on "challenging your thoughts that are telling you you're
having a heart attack," he says. The most severe cases,
however, get medication.

As always with drugs, Dr. Bystritsky says, "There's a

trade-off. You have to weigh the benefits against the hazards." The benefits can be great. These drugs are best for people who, Dr. Bystritsky says, "can't even come close to relaxing and talking about their panic disorder." The right medication (each person responds differently) can stop the attacks within two weeks.

The most commonly prescribed drugs are tricyclic antidepressants like imipramine (Tofranil), monoamine oxidase inhibitors (MAOIs), antidepressants, and alprazolam (Xanax), a Valium cousin. They all work in different ways but do at least one thing: keep the heart from beating too fast. The average treatment lasts for 6 to 12 months, Dr. Sheehan says.

But as beneficial as they are, the trade-offs can be uncomfortable for some, dangerous for others. A major problem with the drugs is relapse. "Even after a year of treatment, 75 to 80 percent of patients will get some recurrence within three to four months after the drug is stopped," Dr. Sheehan says. In some cases, there's a rebound effect: Panic attacks return in even greater numbers and intensity. Gradually reducing the dosage is crucial to successfully withdrawing patients from drugs while preventing rebounding panic attacks. Three-quarters of patients who have to take drugs will need long-term drug therapy, and 25 percent won't be helped regardless of how long they take drugs. Still, a quarter of the patients who do take drugs are helped permanently and won't have to continue them.

Side effects are many: The tricyclics are known to actually cause anxiety in the first days of treatment. The MAOIs react badly with certain foods. Xanax is more sedative, Dr. Bystritsky says, and can be highly addictive and produce severe withdrawal symptoms if the drug is stopped abruptly. However, Dr. Sheehan says, the word *addiction* can be misleading. "To be a truly addictive drug, its use has to produce significant disability," he says. "In contrast, Xanax patients are free of disability. They are actually more able because they no longer have panic attacks."

Overall, though, drugs can give relief so effectively that even psychotherapists sometimes recommend them, if only for a short time. "Someone who's suffering day and night deserves to have some break," Dr. McCullough says.

What to Do
When Panic Strikes

If you're having a panic attack, there's a lot you can do to abort it—or at least to lessen its impact. These tips from the experts may help. The trick is finding one that works for you, then being able to remember it when panic threatens.

Burn up the adrenaline. "The excess adrenaline brought on by a fight-or-flight response is what causes hyperventilation and palpitations," says Christopher McCullough, Ph.D., director of the San Francisco Anxiety and Phobia Recovery Center. To dissipate that adrenaline, try going for a short, brisk walk, or start tensing and relaxing your muscles.

Slow your breathing down. Cool it down to 8 to 12 breaths per minute: Take a deep breath (expand your diaphragm so your stomach pushes out), hold it for a count of four, then exhale slowly.

Don't leave the situation. That encourages the development of phobia, advises Fred Wright, Ed.D., director of education for the University of Pennsylvania Hospital's Center for Cognitive Therapy. If you must leave so you can take a brisk walk, as Dr. McCullough suggests, be sure to come back and face the fear.

Distract yourself. "Distraction is a powerful technique," Dr. Wright says. "Instead of focusing on your physical symptoms, start talking with somebody, or start people-watching, or pay attention to your breathing. You'll notice that almost right away the panic starts fading." Or try splashing cold water on your face or applying a cold washcloth.

CHAPTER 23

Bathe Away Your Winter Blues

If you suffer from fall-to-spring doldrums, you may have seasonal affective disorder. Luckily, daily light baths help up to 80 percent of cases.

Everyone recognizes spring fever, the sudden elation that strikes like a magic spell as the short, dark days of winter give way to the longer, sunny days of spring. Until recently, the opposite condition did not command much attention. But psychological researchers now recognize that some people's winter depressions strike with all the debilitating force of serious emotional problems. Fortunately, this condition can often be self-treated easily and relatively inexpensively without drugs.

Fittingly, the psychiatric term for winter depression is *seasonal affective disorder*, or SAD. Symptoms typically strike from September through February. In addition to the lethargy associated with other forms of depression, SAD symptoms often include irritability, increased appetite, weight gain, increased need for sleep, and in some cases, chronic headache. No one knows how many people experience SAD, but most authorities speculate that it is fairly common. The condition usually begins during a person's twenties and causes significant depression for weeks at a time. About half of SAD sufferers have close relatives with other significant emotional problems. And SAD affects women six times more frequently than men.

Many animal species show profound seasonal behavior changes, for example, hibernation and bird migration. Some researchers speculate that we humans may have similar tendencies. In fact, the lethargy, withdrawal, and weight gain typical in many cases of SAD bear a haunting resemblance to hibernation.

Seasonal behavior changes in animals seem to be related to the light-sensitive pineal gland in the brain. As the days grow shorter, less light energy is transmitted to the brain from the eyes, and the pineal gland releases more of the hormone melatonin. In some animal species, elevated blood levels of melatonin suppress reproduction, which has a significant Darwinian survival advantage. It means that females do not face the increased vulnerability of delivering young during the winter and that offspring are not born during the most challenging time of year. Humans also experience seasonal, light-related melatonin changes, but the hormone's role in SAD, if any, remains unclear.

Do-It-Yourself Phototherapy

Researchers have discovered that some SAD sufferers regularly go south for winter vacations, an almost instinctive form of self-care. The extra day length and greater light intensity temporarily relieve their depression, allowing them to function more normally for a few weeks after they return north.

If Caribbean vacations are not possible, another therapy has also been shown to relieve SAD—daily exposure to a particular form of light. Bright white light that contains the same spectrum of wavelengths as natural sunlight (minus the ultraviolet, which causes sunburn and increases risk of malignant melanoma) can reverse winter depression in the vast majority of SAD sufferers. Relief begins about three days after phototherapy begins, and if phototherapy is discontinued, SAD symptoms typically return within a few weeks.

The apparatus typically recommended for phototherapy is a box about the size of a large television, with six or more fluorescent bulbs inside. For best results, users are advised to sit about three feet away. People with SAD appear to respond best when bathed in this intense full-spectrum light for two or more hours every winter day. Phototherapy is most effective if those who use it glance at the lights periodically to allow more of it to enter their eyes.

Recent studies suggest that phototherapy may be most effective in the morning. About half of SAD sufferers gain significant relief from morning phototherapy sessions, compared with about a third from midday or evening sessions. Those who do not respond to standard phototherapy often find relief after increasing the intensity of the light. However, some evidence suggests that overexposure may cause a maniclike reaction. Such cases usually respond to a reduction in light intensity.

Phototherapy has been shown to treat SAD effectively in up to 80 percent of cases. Michael A. Freeman, M.D., Ph.D., assistant clinical professor of psychiatry, University of California Medical Center in San Francisco, recommends it to his patients. Of course, he also recommends winter vacations to tropical sunny islands. With a diagnosis of SAD, he says, you might even be able to write it off.

CHAPTER 24
Take Control of Epilepsy
By Adrienne Richard

Few people know that many seizures can be blocked or arrested. Here's one woman's success story.

Thirty minutes after the meeting started, Martha felt the first warning signals. An epileptic seizure was about to strike. Instantly she was filled with fear. What could she do? She was alone. Her husband had dropped her off and driven away. She had no way to get home and no time to get there. Her fear and anxiety mounted—signs for her of an oncoming seizure. She knew loss of consciousness and wracking convulsions were drawing near. Desperate, she turned to the only method she could think of, deep relaxing breathing.

"I just concentrated on my breathing," she said later. "I

told myself, think *calm*. And I did. I took one slow, deep breath after another. The seizure rose to a certain point, then stopped as if it couldn't go any further—like it was blocked. Then, after a while, it went away. I don't think anyone at the meeting knew what I was going through."

Martha's ability to arrest a seizure may seem surprising to those unfamiliar with epilepsy, but these days it's more the rule than the exception. Many people with epilepsy now routinely prevent their seizures. Few others realize that self-care methods can consistently block seizures and reduce their severity.

Self-Discovery

I stumbled on self-care for epilepsy by accident. For years, I controlled my massive *grand mal* seizures with medication. But eventually I began to question my reliance on powerful, toxic drugs such as Dilantin and phenobarbital.

A friend introduced me to hatha-yoga. I learned relaxing stretches; deep, diaphragmatic breathing; and the calming, centering effects of meditation. I soon changed my diet—cut down on sugar, protein, and animal fats and increased my consumption of whole grains and other sources of fiber. Very gradually I eliminated my anticonvulsant medication. In the past when I'd dropped my medication, seizures had occurred, but this time I had no problems. I began to feel lighter, more energized. In the 15 years since, I have not had to return to medication, and I've had only two convulsive seizures. From time to time, I have mild, nonconvulsive seizures. I don't find these debilitating but strangely enriching. In addition, I was referred to a progressive neurologist who has encouraged my independence and suggested reading and research that has broadened and deepened my knowledge of this affliction and of myself.

In 1984, I became part of a pilot research project in the Mind/Body Workshop of the Department of Behavioral Medicine at Beth Israel Hospital in Boston under Joan Borysenko, Ph.D., and Herbert Benson, M.D., author of the classic *Relaxation Response*, a guide to scientific meditation. The researchers wondered if the relaxation response might help control seizures. The answer was a resounding yes.

This experience led me to take biofeedback training in the Voluntary Controls Program at the Menninger Foundation in Topeka, Kansas. I also studied the relationship of diet to epilepsy through the Brain-Bio Center in Skillman, New Jersey, and the behavioral aspects of the disease at Boston University. The more I learned, the more clear it became that my self-care methods worked.

But would self-care work for everyone? Perhaps I was a special case. To find out, together with a neurologist and psychiatrist, I designed and led a workshop in self-care for seizures. The majority of participants found our methods helpful, and I continue to present workshops with similar positive results. In Santa Rosa, California, neurologist Joel Reiter, M.D., and Donna Andrews, another self-controlled epileptic, have developed a similar program.

Neurological Malfunction

Epilepsy is no longer regarded as a disease, just as the concept of disease replaced the earlier belief that epilepsy was caused by demonic possession. Today it is called *seizure disorder* to avoid the age-old stigma attached to *epilepsy*.

An epileptic seizure is a symptom of a neurological malfunction in the brain. Somewhere in the brain there is a *discharging lesion*, a minute area that is more electrically excitable than other areas. When this lesion begins to discharge excessively, the surrounding neurons try to contain the excitable neurons. Sometimes they succeed, but when they are overcome, the discharge spreads and a seizure develops. One characteristic of a seizure is the speed at which it comes and goes. Typically, it involves only a few seconds to a few minutes. Afterward, the person may have no memory of the event and may suffer mental confusion while the brain recovers from the overpowering electrical discharge.

Most people are aware of only two types of seizures, *petit mal*, the small lapses of attention, and *grand mal*, which involves convulsions and loss of consciousness. However, there are numerous types of convulsions. The place in the brain where the seizure begins and the areas where it spreads determine the type of seizure. The preliminary warning signs or *aura* of a seizure's onset are also related to the region of the brain where it is focused.

Although we can't see exactly what's happening inside the brain, we can see the unusual body movements, the effects on consciousness, and the changed behavior caused by the malfunctioning cells.

The Medical Workup

A thorough epilepsy workup begins with a visit to a neurologist. The person recounts his or her experiences. Awareness of what has happened is critical. After tests in the office, an electroencephalogram (EEG) in a hospital usually follows. In an EEG, 20 electrodes are glued to the scalp, where they transmit electrical discharges from surface areas of the brain to a polygraph machine that records the discharges as waves, hence "brain waves." If the lesion is in the outer areas of the brain, its excessive firings should show up here. Through a CAT scan of the head, any tumors or injuries may be detected. A complete workup also includes a glucose tolerance test to check whether the seizures are caused by hypoglycemia, excessively low blood sugar.

If the person reports unconscious automatic behavior or strange hallucinatory experiences instead of classic sei-zures, a psychiatric evaluation may also be indicated. These experiences are extremely difficult to diagnose correctly and account for some tragic misdiagnoses in which people are mistakenly committed to mental institutions, then later correctly diagnosed with *partial seizures* or *complex partial seizures*. In each of my workshops, there has been at least one person, often a woman, who still suffers the anger and humiliation of being diagnosed, as one woman termed it, a "mental."

Once epilepsy, or seizure disorder, is diagnosed, the medical treatment of choice is anticonvulsant medication. The doctor prescribes one drug or more from an array of the more than a dozen drugs that affect neurotransmission. The possible side effects of these powerful medications

Types of Seizures

Epileptic seizures fall into two main categories, convulsive and nonconvulsive, which are then described according to characteristic symptoms.

Convulsive

Generalized tonic-clonic (grand mal): This type is characterized by a sudden cry, a fall, rigidity followed by muscle jerks, frothing at the lips, shallow or undetectable breathing, bluish skin, and possible loss of bladder control. The seizure lasts two to five minutes. Afterward, the person may be confused, fatigued, or suffer loss of memory.

Nonconvulsive

Absence (petit mal): This seizure, most common in children, is characterized by a blank stare. Children are unaware of their surroundings during these seizures.

Simple partial (Jacksonian): The person is conscious while jerking begins in the fingers and toes and progresses upward throughout the body.

Simple partial (sensory): The person may hear, see, or sense things that do not exist in the outer world. These may occur alone or as a preliminary symptom of a generalized seizure.

Complex partial (temporal lobe): This type is characterized by a blank stare, chewing motion, and random activity. The person is unaware of his or her surroundings, seems dazed, and may act oddly. Afterward, there is no memory of the seizure.

Atonic (drop attack): A form of childhood seizure in which children lose consciousness for about ten seconds and their legs collapse.

(continued)

Types of Seizures—Continued

Myoclonic: This seizure is characterized by brief, massive muscle jerks.

SOURCE: Adapted from "Epilepsy: Recognition and First Aid," by the Epilepsy Foundation of America, Landover, Maryland.

---

include lack of energy, liver problems, mental fogginess, extreme fatigue, leukemia-like symptoms, and possibly even death. In addition, anticonvulsants inhibit the absorption of calcium, folate, and vitamin D.

The anticonvulsants are undeniably effective in seizure control. More than half of all people with epilepsy achieve complete seizure control with drugs. That was the case with me. Another 15 to 20 percent gain partial control. Just as certain types of seizures are more easily diagnosed, certain types are more easily controlled. Recent research indicates that control within the first two years after diagnosis gives the best indication for staying seizure free in the future. British neurologist E. H. Reynolds says, "There seems little doubt that the drugs play a major role in the high remission rate."

Despite treatment advances, epilepsy remains a mystery. Some people have seizures without showing a trace of injury or seizure focus in the brain. Diagnostic methods cannot penetrate deep into the brain without surgery, and although neurologists' knowledge is growing, it is still limited. Many epilepsy sufferers complain that in the face of uncontrolled seizures, all doctors can do is increase the dosage of medication.

Anyone, Anytime

Anyone can develop epilepsy at any time of life. Most seizures, 75 percent, begin in childhood. "My staring spells," wrote sufferer Kurt Eichenwald in a news magazine, "periods of a few seconds of mental absences, had been going on as long as I could remember." A woman in one of my workshops told how teachers and classmates had ridiculed her as a "space cadet" for her brief petit mal lapses.

For another 25 percent, seizures begin later in life. My grand mal seizures began when I was 21. The Russian writer Dostoyevsky began having seizures at 18. Now that many elderly people are being cared for in nursing facilities, doctors are becoming aware of the incidence of new seizures with advancing age. Sports and automobile head injuries account for many late-onset cases, but the cause of others is unknown (idiopathic). Some people notice curious spells and uncontrollable bursts of odd behavior. These simple or complex partial seizures often go undiagnosed. It's likely that two million North Americans suffer from epileptic seizures of one kind or another. Innumerable others, such as Lewis Carroll, author of *Alice's Adventures in Wonderland*, have only one or two seizures in a lifetime.

Because of its unpredictability, epilepsy is difficult to cope with. The guardian neurons often do their job of containment, but sometimes they don't. The social consequences can be devastating. For two millenia, Western civilization has viewed epilepsy as a curse, or worse, as demonic possession. The stigma continues today, often forcing sufferers to become isolated, fearful of telling others of their condition. When I was first diagnosed, I believed I must never tell anyone. Many people still feel this way. In a few cultures, epilepsy is regarded as a sign of spiritual powers that can be trained and developed to benefit all. But in Western culture, the social stigma makes it doubly difficult to seek help. Most of us find our health care providers through referrals from family and friends. The secrecy of epilepsy closes off this avenue to many sufferers. Most people in my self-care workshops admit they've never talked about their epilepsy with anyone other than their doctor and immediate family.

Self-Care

The importance of self-care for epilepsy can't be overemphasized. Self-care methods enhance the effectiveness of medication, keeping dosage low and increasing the possibility of becoming seizure free and drug free. Self-care can minimize the circumstances conducive to seizures. Those who are particularly drug sensitive or women considering pregnancy can opt for self-care rather than drugs to control seizures. Parents can select methods appropriate for children with epilepsy. And older sufferers can be taught self-care by thoughtful, informed caretakers.

Epilepsy self-care includes attitude, observation, prevention, and intervention.

Attitude. "Only your active participation in seizure control," write Dr. Reiter and Andrews in their book *Taking Control of Your Epilepsy* (available from Epilepsy Research Program, 550 Doyle Park Drive, Santa Rosa, CA 95045), "will enable you to reach your optimum level of wellness." The first step, they say, is "making the decision to take control."

This is easier for some than others. To build and maintain the kind of attitude it takes to control seizures, you need a supportive environment. In the workshops I lead, participants become a support system for one another.

Equally important is your commitment to the decision to take control. I have workshop participants write on sheets from prescription pads, "I want my brain cells to act calmly and normally. I will do everything I can to help my brain cells act calmly and normally." Each then signs his or her name on the physician signature line.

One consequence of this decision is giving up the special status epilepsy provides, either as a victim or a recipient of special privileges. You can no longer say, "I can't. I'm epileptic." You have decided to be a person—who incidentally has seizures. While it may sound easy, most find it is not.

Observation. To learn what conditions and circumstances make them seizure prone, epileptics must observe their physical and emotional responses closely. One of my two grand mal seizures during the past 15 years occurred after a week of fatigue, extreme tension, overexposure to heat and sun, and a glass of wine every night in a setting that allowed no time or space to take care of myself and do my relaxing exercises. I learned from the experience what triggers my massive seizures.

Every time a seizure breaks through, ask yourself these questions:

- Was I under emotional stress? What were the reasons for the stress (for example, work, relationships, placing unreasonable demands on yourself)?
- Was I under physical stress (for example, fatigue, illness, menstruation, too much sun)?
- How balanced was my diet?

Dr. Reiter and Andrews recommend a "seizure log," a brief summary of each seizure and the conditions surrounding it. My workshop participants say they find such logs helpful.

Anyone with seizure disorder must also observe his or her aura, the early warning signs that a seizure is about to begin. Aura signs may be strange experiences: the feeling of being spacey and light-headed; detection of odd smells, sights, and sounds; "surges" of feeling through the neck and head; nervousness and hyperactivity; increased intuitive powers; or many other odd sensations.

Most epileptics learn to recognize their early warning signs with a little training. One man told me he couldn't observe his aura, but that his wife could. She tells him when he gets irritable and erratic. This mood swing indicates high risk and the need to care for himself—getting rest, eating well, releasing tension, and avoiding emotional and physical stressors until he returns to normal.

Prevention. Stress and tension are notable precipitants of seizures. Some people find they survive stressful weeks, then have Saturday seizures or vacation seizures once the stress lets up. It's important to prevent the accumulation of physical and neurophysical tensions. Release stress and tension with regular exercise 20 to 30 minutes a day.

Any form of gentle but vigorous exercise releases tension and improves mood. Fast walking, low-impact aerobics, and yogic stretches are all excellent. (Training for competition increases tension.)

I recommend progressive muscle relaxation (PMR). In a study conducted at the University of Minnesota School of Nursing, 75 percent of those who practiced PMR every other day largely controlled their seizures.

Progressive
Muscle Relaxation

This series of exercises progresses from the feet to the head and takes about ten minutes. Its effectiveness comes from alternately tensing and relaxing each muscle group. Tense, hold, and relax for about five seconds each.

1. Curl toes tightly. Hold. Relax. Rest.
2. Flex the feet. Hold. Relax. Rest.
3. Tighten the calves. Hold. Relax. Rest.
4. Tense the thighs. Hold. Relax. Rest.
5. Tighten the buttocks. Hold. Relax. Rest.
6. Tighten the lower back. Hold. Relax. Rest.
7. Tighten the abdomen. Hold. Relax. Rest.
8. Tense the upper chest. Hold. Relax. Rest.
9. Tense the upper back muscles. Hold. Relax. Rest.
10. Clench the fists. Hold. Relax. Rest.
11. Extend the fingers and flex the wrists. Hold. Relax. Rest.
12. Tighten the forearms. Hold. Relax. Rest.
13. Tighten the upper arms. Hold. Relax. Rest.
14. Lift the shoulders gently toward the ears. Hold. Let them drop.
15. Wrinkle the forehead. Hold. Relax. Rest.
16. Squeeze your eyes shut. Hold. Relax. Rest.
17. Drop your chin, letting your mouth open wide. Hold. Relax. Rest.
18. Lift the shoulders gently and then pull them down as if you had weights in your hands. Let them rise to their natural position.

Do head rolls and shoulder shrugs—slowly and gently—to release neck and shoulder tension and increase circulation to the head. Deep relaxation can be achieved through deep diaphragmatic breathing. Dr. Benson uses this type of breathing to induce the *relaxation response* characteristic of many forms of meditation. Deep diaphragmatic breathing is simple but takes practice:

1. Lie on the floor and place one hand on your abdomen and one on your upper chest.
2. Inhale deeply so your abdomen expands like a balloon and your upper chest remains still. Exhale, feeling the abdomen fall.
3. Close your eyes and focus your attention on the rise and fall of your abdomen as you breathe. When your mind wanders, gently return your attention to your breath.

Breathe deeply for 20 minutes a day. Most people find deep relaxation immensely refreshing.

One note of caution: Deep diaphragmatic breathing may cause seizures in some people. I believe the reason has to do with the release of accumulated tension. If this happens to you more than once or twice, discontinue deep relaxation. Others, including myself, use deep diaphragmatic breathing as seizure intervention.

Diet and nutritional supplements are particularly important for epilepsy sufferers. A nutritionally sound diet enhances health and increases energy and alertness. There are two special diets helpful with seizures—the ketogenic and hypoglycemic diets. Both require a physician's guidance. Generally, however, a high-fiber, low-fat, low-sugar diet with moderate amounts of protein helps build resistance to seizures.

To increase the fiber in your diet, eat plenty of whole grains such as whole wheat, oat or wheat bran, and brown rice, fresh fruits with skins, and steamed, baked, or quickly sauteed fresh vegetables. You can decrease fat by eating more fish and skinless chicken, cooking in water or broth rather than fat, and baking trimmed meats on a drip rack.

Avoid refined sugars, honey, and syrups as much as possible.

Nutritional supplements can be important for epileptic sufferers. Anticonvulsant medications inhibit the absorption of calcium, folate, and vitamin D. Supplementing with calcium carbonate, vitamin D, and vitamin B complex is important. According to Carl Pfeiffer, M.D., at New Jersey's Brain-Bio Center, vitamins B_6 and B_{12} and the minerals manganese and magnesium improve brain function and inhibit seizures. However, B_6 interferes with the effectiveness of Dilantin. If you take this drug, keep your daily B_6 intake below 25 milligrams.

Avoid the following substances:

- Alcohol puts certain brain cells "to sleep," causes drowsiness, and taxes the liver.
- Caffeine gives glucose a fast boost, then a fast drop.
- Artificial sweeteners, such as NutraSweet, have been associated with seizures.
- Nicotine interferes with the blood's oxygen supply.
- Lead causes seizures in children.
- Aluminum, often found in deodorants and buffered aspirin, is thought to impair brain function.
- Pesticides, some of them, can cause seizures on skin contact. If you must use pesticides, wear protective clothing.

Intervention

Few people realize that most, and in some cases all, seizures can be blocked or arrested. A noted study of inhibiting grand mal seizures was reported by neurologist Robert Efron, M.D., in the mid-1950s. He found one woman's seizures were always preceded by a certain odor. He gave her essence of jasmine to sniff when she detected the telltale aroma. The jasmine effectively blocked her seizures, and she was able to stop her medication. Later, Dr. Efron taught the woman to associate the jasmine smell with the mental image of a silver bracelet. When she smelled the preseizure aroma, she pictured the silver bracelet, which triggered the jasmine to block the seizure.

Dr. Efron's experiment underscores the most important elements of intervention: observing the aura, or preliminary signs, knowing the correct preventive image or action, and taking action in time.

More recently, neurologist Paul Pritchard, M.D., led a team that recorded the acts and mental images of seven people who successfully blocked their seizures. Several used physical movement while others used prayer, meditation, concentration, or imagery. One man who visualized a fishing trip had an EEG that measured his ability to block seizure impulse for as long as three minutes while visualizing.

Certain types of seizures are easier to block than others. Brief lapses of consciousness and complex partial seizures are considered difficult to block, but some people say they can do it. One man in my workshops said he instructed his secretary to shout at him if she noticed him lapsing into unconsciousness. When she did, he was able to remain conscious and remember the spell for the first time in his life. Martha, who was able to block her seizure at the meeting described earlier, uses deep diaphragmatic breathing when a grand mal seizure threatens.

Learn to use intervention effectively:

- Discover what images or actions work for you. Deeply relaxing images are helpful for some, while others need to be startled by a shout and/or a shake.
- Practice, so you know what to do when the time comes.
- Carefully observe your preliminary warning signs.
- Use your intervention method the moment you notice any warning sign.

Other methods also help control seizures. Biofeedback can control brain waves and block seizures, but it takes training and machinery. Psychotherapy can alleviate deep tensions that contribute to seizure conditions. But the methods described here are the most helpful and accessible:

- Take charge of yourself.
- Observe the conditions and circumstances when seizures occur.

- Alleviate or change these conditions or circumstances with preventive measures.
- Find a method of intervention that works for you and use it when you need it.

A year has passed since Martha first used deep diaphragmatic breathing to block a threatened seizure. Now she meditates at bedtime, practices deep breathing and gentle exercises, and has gained much greater control of her life.

PART V:
MEDICAL TESTS AND
YOUR HEALTH

Flash Reports

MAKING CHLAMYDIA
DETECTION EASIER

Genital warts may be the most commonly *diagnosed* sexually transmitted disease (STD), but chlamydia is the most common. Chlamydia starts with transmission of bacteria, usually *Chlamydia trachomatis*, during intercourse. In half of infected women and one-quarter of infected men, no symptoms occur—doctors call chlamydia the silent STD—so the disease often goes undiagnosed. If symptoms do develop, the most common are a genital discharge and pain during urination. Untreated, it can lead to pelvic inflammatory disease, ectopic pregnancy (gestation outside the uterus, such as in a fallopian tube), and infertility.

Until recently, the only way to detect the disease was to take a sample of genital secretions and grow the bacteria. The old test cost up to $50 and often failed because chlamydia bacteria don't grow well in laboratories.

New chlamydia tests are cheaper, faster, and equally (some doctors even say more) accurate. The new tests can be done in a doctor's office, with results in 30 minutes, and cost about $25.

As with a Pap smear, the doctor swabs a sample from the cervix. The sample is then placed in a tube, and a liquid that helps identify chlamydia bacteria is added. The liquid is then poured onto a specially treated disk, which produces a plus sign if chlamydia is present.

Although most doctors agree these new tests are an improvement, the tests share a limitation with older ones: The doctor may not swab enough cells to yield accurate results.

It's better, doctors say, to prevent chlamydia in the first place by using a condom or diaphragm or practicing monogamy.

LUNG CANCER TEST OF THE FUTURE

An experimental lung cancer test may be able to detect the disease at least two years before it's perceptible on x-rays, a preliminary study suggests. That would make the test a bona fide breakthrough, if further research confirms its usefulness. Right now, lung cancer is almost impossible to detect before severe and often fatal damage has been done to the body.

The test uses monoclonal antibodies—molecules similar to disease-fighting substances produced by the body. Since lung cancer sheds cancer cells into the sputum, or saliva, the test is performed by putting the monoclonal antibodies into a saliva sample. The monoclonal antibodies seek out and latch onto so-called target sites on any lung cancer cells that are present, pinpointing the cells long before other tests can identify them.

In a recently published study, the test was used on sputum specimens collected from a previous Johns Hopkins University study conducted from 1973 to 1981. The test correctly diagnosed lung cancer in 20 of 22 patients who later developed the disease. It also found no indication of lung cancer in 35 of 40 people who later did not get the disease.

"I frankly think this is a very exciting development in the detection and treatment of all cancers," says James Mulshine, M.D., head of the biotherapy section at the National Cancer Institute. He says that clinical trials of the test will begin in a year, but that solid justification for its widespread use is at least five to ten years away.

FINDING FOOD ALLERGIES

Is your nose stuffed up or runny year-round? Foods, *not* pollen or pets, may be the cause, says Dutch researcher Zdenek Pelikan, M.D.

Dr. Pelikan studied 142 patients with nasal problems. Some said they had noticed foods seemed to cause their symptoms; others did not. For a week, they ate a low-allergy diet. Then they took capsules of extracts of possible symptom-causing foods. (They weren't told what food extracts they were getting.) Their reactions were followed for 56 hours.

The results? Eighty-seven percent of those who'd suspected a food-nose link, and 57 percent who hadn't, reacted. Some had sneezing and a runny nose, which peaked within two hours of eating. Others had a delayed response, mostly stuffiness and nasal itching, that peaked at seven to nine hours.

This study didn't reveal which foods caused the most problems. Cheese, eggs, milk, peanuts, chocolate, beer, wine, shrimp, and spices were among those tested, since they are common allergy-producing foods.

CHAPTER 25

Update on Osteoporosis Screening

Experts offer advice on who should and who shouldn't be tested for bone problems.

Blood pressure testing is no big deal. Strap on a cuff, and a few minutes later you may be on the road to detecting—and blocking—a dangerous case of hypertension. Cholesterol tests are nearly as easy and useful. But what about bone densitometry, the high-tech tests that are intended to detect osteoporosis? Like x-rays, these tests are noninvasive—no surgery required—and some involve only low doses of radiation. But the price is steep, from $35 to $350. And experts caution that, for many people, they may not be worth the money or effort.

That's not to say osteoporosis isn't a serious problem. It is, especially for older women. In the five to ten years after menopause, when estrogen levels plummet, calcium leaches from the bones at an accelerated rate. The result: a porous bone condition that can weaken the skeletal frame to the point where a slight injury—or even an abrupt move—can cause a fracture. The spine and hip are especially vulnerable. Spinal fractures can cause "dowager's hump" and chronic pain; hip fractures can be crippling and sometimes fatal. So there is good reason for concern.

The question is, can early detection prevent some of the serious consequences of the disease? And is there a place for screening (testing and retesting) of all women beginning at age 35, when bone loss theoretically begins?

Premenopausal Screening Debate

Some say yes. Over the past few years, the bone densi-ty testing business has boomed: Doctors' offices, hospi-tals, and walk-in clinics offering the examinations have proliferated.

When a private osteoporosis diagnostic center in New York City was contacted, the woman who answered the telephone encouraged the caller to hurry in. "You're in your midthirties? You're absolutely the perfect age! Come get tested so you'll know how dense your bones are now, at their peak, and to learn what you can do to prevent osteoporosis!" She went on to explain that the fee for the bone density test is $200 and the consultation another $100, and that insurance probably wouldn't cover most of the costs. "Would you like to schedule an appointment?" The caller declined.

The National Osteoporosis Foundation—along with many physicians who specialize in bone densitometry—rejects the idea of mass screening. They are especially critical of testing centers that invite virtually anyone in for a bone scan.

"There's almost no reason for a woman who is premeno-pausal to get a bone density test," says B. Lawrence Riggs, M.D., adviser to the National Osteoporosis Foundation. "There's not a lot of bone loss prior to menopause," he explains.

There are a few exceptions. Younger women with hor-monal disorders, premature menopause, anorexia, oopho-rectomy (removal of the ovaries), or unexplained fracturing may have osteoporosis. "These are women with disease, not healthy, normal women," says Diane Meier, M.D., codirector of Mount Sinai Hospital's Osteoporosis Program in New York. The test can help diagnose the problem and lead to treatment. Some osteoporosis centers—such as the one mentioned above—claim that the results of a bone density test can draw a young woman's attention to prob-lems with her lifestyle, such as a lack of dietary calcium. But most physicians disagree. "I think it's an expensive way to entice a woman to drink more milk," says Harvard radiologist Ferris Hall, M.D.

Finally, a few purveyors of the test argue that a measurement of bone mass at age 35 will provide a baseline for measurements in the future. But other physicians concur that a single figure for a younger woman probably wouldn't have much meaning.

Test Shortcomings

Sophisticated though these bone tests may be (see "Comparing the Tests"), they do have their shortcomings: First, a single test can't predict the rate of bone loss. And even if tests are repeated, they often are not precise enough to detect small but significant changes in bone density. Quality control must be very strict, and tests must be repeated frequently to detect small losses.

Second, while the tests do indicate bone density at the sites they measure—and bone density is the best indication of your likelihood of fracturing—the tests are poor at predicting the most serious fractures, those of the hip.

These are some of the reasons that the American College of Physicians last year issued a position paper calling for more research into bone densitometry before using it on a wider population. "Right now, you get a value back and you can't tell what it means, except that you're probably at somewhat greater risk or less risk than average. That's not very helpful," says the paper's author, Steven Cummings, M.D. For similar reasons, the U.S. Public Health Service has also called for further study of bone density assessment techniques. Until then, they've recommended that Medicare not reimburse for most densitometry tests. If private insurers follow their lead, fewer people at any age will get tested.

Despite its shortcomings, however, bone densitometry is useful for certain people. According to the American College of Physicians and the National Osteoporosis Foundation, the best candidate is a woman who has reached menopause, who has several risk factors for the disease, and who may be considering estrogen replacement therapy. (Estrogen replacement therapy is the preferred preventive for osteoporosis in the menopausal years. Some physicians may also recommend calcium supplements.)

Comparing the Tests

Ordinary x-rays don't reveal osteoporosis until virtually a third of bone is gone. In recent years, scientists have developed—and are still developing—better ways to measure bone density. These are the most common.

Single photon absorptiometry (SPA). This test measures the density of bones in the forearm or heel. The bone is penetrated by a narrow beam of photons from a radioactive source. Radiation dosage is quite low, under 10 millirems (a standard chest x-ray is 60 to 100 millirems). Costs run from $35 to $120. When it was first developed, SPA caught on fast, and many new osteoporosis centers offered it as their diagnostic test for menopausal women. But medical experts now agree that SPA's uses are more limited and that it's not a good predictor of bone loss at the most troublesome sites, the hips and the spine. It is considered most useful in patients over 75 and in measuring large changes in bone density due to medical treatments.

Dual-photon absorptiometry (DPA). It's similar to SPA, except that the radioactive source produces two beams, for a more precise measurement. Unlike SPA, it can also be used to measure the hip, the spine, and other skeletal sites. Radiation exposure is also low, about 30 millirems. It costs from $50 to $300. This test is considered most appropriate for middle-aged women, because it does measure the hip and spine. It's less useful than CAT scans for patients over 75 or for patients who have calcium deposits or bone degeneration around the spine.

Quantitative computerized axial tomography (CAT). Here x-rays are used to generate cross-sectional images of vertebrae and other sites. The radia-
(continued)

Comparing the Tests—Continued

tion exposure is larger than the first two methods:
from 100 to 1,000 millirems, averaging 300 millirems.
It costs from $100 to $350. CAT scans can be useful for
patients of any age, but because of the high radiation
exposure, repeated tests are a problem.

Dual-energy radiography. Still in development,
this test promises better precision, lower radiation,
and less cost.

Others agree that bone tests make the most sense for
menopausal women who have one major or several
"broadly based" risk factors for osteoporosis. The broadly
based risk factors include being white or Asian, being thin
and petite, having a family history of osteoporosis, having
a low calcium intake, smoking, social alcohol use, never
having had children, and having a sedentary lifestyle.

The major risk factors, says Dr. Riggs, include certain
diseases, including hormonal and gastrointestinal disorders, premature menopause, alcoholism, and treatment
with certain medications and hormones (check with your
physician). Of course, even if you do have several of the
minor risk factors, the test is mainly of value if you are
considering estrogen therapy. If you and your physician
have already determined that hormonal therapy is not for
you—perhaps you have contraindications, such as a family
history of cancer or risk of stroke—the test is unnecessary.
Likewise, if you and your physician have already determined that hormonal therapy is in your best interest—
regardless of the test results—there's no point in doing the
test. In either case, the test results won't affect your course
of treatment. Bone densitometry is useful only if there is
some question whether you would benefit from estrogen
replacement therapy.

If a woman chooses not to take estrogen after her first
test or the test shows minimal bone loss, Dr. Riggs recom-

mends retesting in three or four years. If the second test shows substantial bone loss, he says, estrogen replacement therapy can be reconsidered.

If you think you're a candidate for a bone density test, talk to your doctor. The next step will be to find a teaching hospital or a reputable clinic where a complete medical evaluation is offered along with the tests. "What you need," says Louis Avioli, M.D., "is a staff of physicians and medics who can advise you."

And remember: With osteoporosis, prevention—not detection—gives you the best edge.

CHAPTER 26
Calming Those Pretest Nerves

People fall into two categories when faced with anxiety. Identify your own coping style and avoid medical test jitters.

When Sylvia left her doctor's office, she was shaking. She leaned against the wall in the corridor, took a deep breath, and tried to calm down. Her doctor had discovered a small but suspicious lump in her breast and had recommended that she go right into a hospital for a mammogram.

She couldn't stop wondering: Will the test hurt? Will I have to disrobe in front of a roomful of doctors and technicians? And, most painful of all, what if it's cancer?

It wasn't cancer. The test was negative. But the anxiety it produced was real—and typical. For a lot of people, dread of a medical test is often more painful than the test itself. And almost any test can induce sweat and tears— from a simple blood test to a CAT scan.

Harvard psychiatrist Lawrence Hartmann, M.D., says

that anxiety over medical testing can be divided into two kinds. First, there's the nervous anticipation of the testing procedure, also called pretest jitters. And second, there's the fear that the test results might reveal a serious medical problem.

Once you've pinpointed the root of your anxiety, you may find it helpful to identify your personal coping style. Most people are either sensitizers or repressors, therapists say. Sensitizers are people who submerge themselves in the problem at hand; they find solace through speaking with others and gathering facts. Repressors need to distract themselves from the anxiety-producing thoughts; they keep busy with other pursuits to avoid confronting their fears. Each coping style has its advantages and shortcomings. Sensitizers tend to be more anxiety prone because they often exaggerate or magnify a problem, says Richard Wessler, Ph.D., chairman of the Psychology Department at Pace University in New York. Repressors tend to minimize or play down stressful events, often denying the degree to which they are a problem.

According to Joseph P. Bush, Ph.D., a psychologist at Virginia Commonwealth University in Richmond, who has conducted extensive research on stressful medical tests, most people fall somewhere between the sensitizer and repressor categories. "It's important, though," he says, "to find out which way you lean so you can figure out how you can best cope with your anxiety."

Think about how you coped the last time you faced a stressful situation: Did you want to know all the facts, or did you try to ignore them? Then, suggests Dr. Bush, ask yourself what would make you feel more comfortable about an upcoming test—watching a videotape of the medical procedure or a relaxation videotape? Sensitizers are likely to want to see the former; repressors are apt to go for the latter.

Broad-Spectrum Coping

Once you know what's provoking your pretest anxiety— and which coping style suits you best—you're ready to tackle tension head on. First, relax.

Take a brisk walk. Aerobic exercise leads to significant reductions in anxiety, according to a recent study from the University of Wisconsin. And long walks—whether they're vigorous enough to be aerobic or not—can serve as great opportunities to share your fears and feelings with someone.

Go for deep relaxation. A variety of stress reduction techniques are available—from meditation to progressive muscle relaxation to having a warm soak in a tub. In general, they cost you little (like relaxation tapes) or nothing (like visualizing yourself in peaceful surroundings). And, as research shows, they all may help reduce your stress and anxiety.

Except in extreme sensitizer or repressor cases, you can probably benefit from some aspects of both coping styles.

Open up. If you're concerned about a proposed diagnostic test—and especially if that test is designed to detect a life-threatening illness—your first response may be to withdraw. In fact, sharing your concerns with a caring person may be a better coping response. In a study conducted by psychiatrist Paul Horton, M.D., 86 percent of the participants chose "being with someone else" as their most frequent choice when seeking solace.

Talking through your fears can help you put them into perspective. It can also give you a sense of control of your situation. Just know whom you're talking with, say the experts. People who are misinformed—or who've had negative experiences themselves—can fan your fears. Unless you're speaking to someone who has had a successful experience with a test—and your doctor may be able to help you get in touch with someone who has—avoid talking about test specifics.

A good option: You can talk to a hospital social worker or psychiatric counselor. Most hospitals have them, and they're trained to help people deal with the fear of testing.

If you don't want to talk to anybody, at least talk to yourself. Keeping a diary before and after your test is a good way to talk out your fears and show how you may be distorting reality.

Get lost. The experts agree that, to some extent, distraction can also help alleviate anxiety. They recommend trying some project that you can lose yourself in for a while. Clean out a closet, knit a sweater, build a birdhouse, write a poem. Mark your calendar for when you'll finish the project, so you'll have a date to think about other than your test date. If you're not interested in projects, you can try less ambitious forms of distraction—like watching television or reading a book (happy endings only!).

Dealing with Pretest Jitters

To short-circuit anxiety before and during the test, the experts recommend the following strategies.

Ask questions. If you're more of a sensitizer than a repressor, you'll probably feel better if you ask: Why do I need this test? What exactly will be done to me? How long will the procedure take? What are the alternatives? How will the results affect treatment of my condition? The answers may not only reduce your fears but give you more control over the situation.

Dr. Hartmann says that it's especially important to ask your "secret" questions, those you're most reluctant to ask because you're afraid of the answers. Laid on the table, these questions (and their answers) may not seem as terrible as you thought. Bottled up inside, your fears may continue to grow out of proportion to reality.

Carolyn Messner, social work supervisor at Cancer Care in New York City, suggests that you go to your doctor's office with a written list of questions. "If you don't have anyone with you, bring a tape recorder," she says. "When you're anxious, your concentration tends to be slack, and you'll probably walk out remembering little of what was said."

Search for peace of mind. If your doctor hasn't answered your questions to your satisfaction or hasn't convinced you of the necessity of a particular test, get a second opinion. Asking for another opinion doesn't show a lack of trust in your physician. Most doctors welcome such a request because the other opinion usually reinforces the original diagnosis and makes the patient feel more comfortable with the decision.

Don't delay. Putting off a necessary test prolongs stress and may increase your risk if you really do have a disease. So once you're sure that you need a test, schedule it as soon as possible and let your doctor know that you want the results quickly. Matthew Loscalzo, director of the Social Work Behavioral Team at Memorial Sloan-Kettering Cancer Center in New York City, recommends that you ask your physician for a specific time and day when you can call for test results.

Schedule it early. If you have the test first thing in the morning, you won't spend the day dreading the appointed hour. For many tests, an early appointment also increases the chances that you'll get results the same day and thus avoid a possibly restless night.

Sneak a preview. If becoming more familiar with your test makes you feel more at ease, take advantage of the information available through many hospitals and doctors. They often have pamphlets and even videotapes describing procedures.

Most hospitals also allow you to check out the facilities and talk to either the people who'll be involved in your procedure or, at least, professionals familiar with the test. (It may not always be possible to find out ahead of time who'll be there for the procedure.)

Seeing the facilities and equipment, especially exotic machines like CAT scanners, can make them less threatening. Dr. Hartmann remembers the case of a patient who chose not to preview her upcoming magnetic resonance imaging (MRI) test, a painless procedure that involves no known risks or side effects. Upon being placed into the imaging machine, she panicked. "Being put into a small space or an apparatus that looks like a coffin taps fears for many people," Dr. Hartmann says.

Visualize. If your anxiety is mild, try this visualization technique: Close your eyes and imagine yourself going through the medical test, step by step. Imagine the sounds, smells, sights, sensations of the whole ordeal. (You needn't dwell, though, on any details that make you extremely uneasy.) Then see yourself coming through it all with flying colors. After several tries at this visualization, you should feel much less anxious.

If you're extremely upset, don't visualize the testing itself. Instead, imagine having successfully completed the test and being in pleasant, safe surroundings.

Observe the test-day "rules." Make test day as normal as possible while still obeying medical instructions regarding diet and other preparations. Avoid stimulants, such as caffeine. Leave as much time for the test as you can, and by all means don't schedule anything else for that day. You may not, for example, be up for a business meeting after a cardiac stress test.

Bring someone with you, if not for emotional support then at least to drive you home. Anesthesia can take a while to wear off. Don't bring children. They might upset not only you but those around you as well.

Bring a tape player. Relaxation need not end when you leave home. If you have a soothing music or relaxation tape, you may be able to listen to it during the test. Under most circumstances these days, people are allowed to bring a tape player into tests done in a hospital—even tests involving radiation. Earphones can usually be used as well, except for tests involving the head or using magnetic fields. Just make sure you ask permission first.

Handling Post-Test Blues

If the time before the test is anxiety producing, the time between the test and the reporting of the results can be even more so. Many people say that the time spent waiting for test results was the worst experience they ever had.

It helps to realize that things are now out of your hands. This may be difficult for people who are used to making decisions and having a lot of control in their lives, but it's essential for peace of mind.

Here are two steps you can take—in addition to the techniques mentioned above—to help minimize posttest strain:

• Avoid scheduling a test at the end of a week, especially on a Friday. There are better things to do with a weekend than spend it agonizing over test results. The earlier in the week you schedule, the more likely you are to get results that same week.

- Change your worries into a plan of action. Consider the worst reasonable thing that could happen, and make a plan for how you would go from there. The point here is not to dwell on the negative, says Dr. Wessler, but to learn to cope by preparing for what you can do next.

It's also good to remember that most people who have anxiety responses to a medical test are perfectly sane. "The anxiety they experience," says Loscalzo, "is usually the result of negative self-defeating fears and fantasies about the test and its potential results."

CHAPTER 27

A New Look at B$_{12}$ Deficiency

Current methods miss many who are truly lacking in this crucial nutrient.

No energy? Appetite under par? Can't remember the very thing you promised yourself you wouldn't forget?

Vague complaints like these can suggest a wide variety of health problems, including a B$_{12}$ deficiency. But it's a rare blood test that detects such a deficiency. So, say doctors, B$_{12}$ injections are hardly ever warranted.

Now two new studies challenge that point of view. They suggest that for some people with "normal" blood tests, B$_{12}$ supplementation may be more than a shot in the dark. It may offer relief from a wide variety of complaints, including fatigue, memory loss, and even incontinence.

A Vital Vitamin

What exactly is B_{12}? Otherwise known as cobalamin, it's important for normal growth, blood formation, and a healthy nervous system. Vitamin B_{12} plays an integral part in the formation of blood cells. Without it, red blood cell production decreases. The result of this B_{12} bombshell: anemia (which starves the body of oxygen, causing tiredness), bleeding, or infections.

Also, the vitamin quite literally keeps you from losing your nerve. B_{12} helps produce myelin, the protective coating that surrounds the nerves, much like rubber encases electrical wiring. Without myelin, nerves slowly deteriorate, causing a potpourri of neuropsychiatric problems. Your feet can become numb and tingle. You can have trouble walking or difficulty feeling the floor. The nerve damage can bring on the more subtle mental changes of the B_{12} blues—depression, confusion, and loss of memory.

Surprisingly, B_{12} deficiency usually isn't the result of ingesting too little B_{12} (the Recommended Dietary Allowance is only three micrograms, which most people easily get with their normal diet). More often, it's caused by an absorption problem. With aging, the stomach can lose its ability to produce intrinsic factor, a substance that allows B_{12} to be absorbed in the small intestine. That's why people who are deficient in B_{12} usually need to take shots—to circumvent the digestive system.

In Search of B_{12}

The question is, how could some people who are presumed not to have B_{12} deficiency actually benefit from a B_{12} boost?

To understand, we must first look at how doctors determine B_{12} deficiency. Many physicians expect B_{12} deficiency to cause blood abnormalities long before it causes nerve damage (except in rare instances). So they often discount B_{12} deficiency if tests show normal blood, says Robert H. Allen, M.D., director of hematology at the University of Colorado Health Sciences Center.

In a study, however, Dr. Allen and his colleagues looked

at 323 patients who suffered from B_{12} deficiency and discovered that 141 had symptoms of nerve damage. Contrary to traditional medical thinking, 40 of the 141 patients (28 percent) were found not to have the expected blood abnormalities.

"I think the most important thing this study shows is that many of the standard teachings about B_{12} deficiency are wrong," says Dr. Allen.

In another new study, from the University of Southern California (USC), 23 of 70 patients with B_{12} deficiency (33 percent) didn't have noticeable blood problems. Ralph Carmel, M.D., author of the study, concludes, "The experience at our hospital suggests that true [B_{12}] deficiency is more common than is currently appreciated."

Another part of the problem, doctors say, is the way B_{12} is measured. The standard test for B_{12} was modified in 1978. The reason was that the test was discovered to react to some compounds that are similar to but are not B_{12}, creating falsely high B_{12} readings. "A lot of cases of B_{12} deficiency were missed because of that," says William S. Beck, M.D., professor of medicine at Harvard Medical School and director of hematology research at Massachusetts General Hospital. "Testing methods were corrected, so that's no longer a problem."

Now the problem seems to be what doctors expect to find when they measure B_{12} serum levels (in the blood)— the first test for determining deficiency. The normal range for B_{12} in the blood is about 200 to 900 picograms per milliliter. Most medical textbooks teach that true deficiency is based on finding serum B_{12} levels of less than 100. But in Dr. Allen's study, 18 of the 40 deficient patients without blood abnormalities had levels between 100 and 200 (slightly low), and two actually had normal B_{12} readings. This is why their B_{12} deficiency could easily have been overlooked. Slightly low or low normal levels could have been dismissed as lab errors, as not worth investigating in this age of medical cost consciousness (especially when the expected anemia or other blood abnormalities weren't present). In the USC study, only 45 of the 70 deficient patients had the very low serum levels expected with B_{12} deficiency.

Also, though Dr. Allen and others use 200 picograms per milliliter as a benchmark for B_{12} deficiency, the exact number can vary from lab to lab.

The bright note to all this is that B_{12} deficiency now seems to become apparent in lab tests at an earlier stage than many doctors have thought. Leading researchers now believe that many cases of B_{12} deficiency can be detected before they even begin to cause serious damage. And that's important because the quicker the problem is caught, the more likely it is to be reversed.

Surprising Symptoms

And the B_{12} deficiency symptoms may be more numerous than many experts realize. In Dr. Allen's study, the patients had reported a total of 212 problems related to nerve damage, including abnormal gait, impaired touch or pain perception, decreased reflexes, and memory loss. After receiving B_{12} injections, 119 of the problems were completely resolved and 59 were partially resolved. In all, no improvement was shown for only 8 of the problems attributed to lack of B_{12}. And all of the participants who completed the study showed at least some progress.

The list of problems that disappeared after B_{12} injections was not only long but also included some surprises—hallucinations, eye disorders, and incontinence. "Most people would never associate incontinence with B_{12} deficiency," says Dr. Allen.

"How common is this? I can't put a number on it, and I wouldn't say it was very common. But I recently read an article in the *New England Journal of Medicine* about incontinence, and it didn't even mention B_{12} deficiency as a possible cause."

Victor Herbert, M.D., professor of medicine at Mount Sinai and Veterans Administration Bronx Medical Centers and a leading B_{12} researcher, says he and others wrote about the association between B_{12} deficiency and problems such as incontinence way back in the 1950s.

Why these symptoms are seldom linked to B_{12} deficiency nowadays is illustrated by Dr. Allen's study. Though there was a control group, it's difficult to know how many of these patients would have improved without B_{12} injections—and therefore how many symptoms weren't caused by deficiency. Many of these psychological problems are vague, waxing and waning, so they're hard to measure scientifically. These technical problems have long vexed B_{12} researchers and may be why symptoms that Dr. Herbert wrote about more than 30 years ago are still not included in some medical review articles.

Testing for B_{12}

So in light of all this, when should you have a B_{12} serum test?

- Consider being tested as soon as you exhibit unexplained nerve or blood problems of the kind that are seen in B_{12} deficiency. If your serum B_{12} level is below 300, Dr. Allen recommends an additional test—just now available commercially through several national labs. This test measures blood elements called metabolites. These elements (specifically methylmalonic acid and total homocysteine) increase in blood when B_{12} is deficient. If your symptoms strongly suggest B_{12} deficiency, Dr. Allen believes this additional test should be done even when the serum B_{12} level is above 300.
- Consider being tested at age 60, whether or not you show signs of deficiency, Dr. Herbert says. If your serum level is low or low normal, you should have another screening within three to six months. Based on that, you can determine with your doctor whether or not you need B_{12} supplementation.

The Placebo Effect

Though he believes that more research like Dr. Allen's is needed, Dr. Beck raised an intriguing question in his editorial accompanying the study: "Could it be that the many [B_{12}] injections given over the years for vague symptoms were in fact justified?" Perhaps. But though there is much confusion in the B_{12} field, experts agree on this point: There is no biological reason that B_{12} should give you a

The Trouble with Tempeh

Vegetarians had long thought they could get sufficient vitamin B_{12} in tempeh, a type of fermented soybean. The tempeh culture itself didn't produce B_{12}, but it was believed to carry bacterial microorganisms that did. But experts have concluded that's not so.

"Until recently, most tempeh manufacturers would not only make B_{12} claims on the nutritional panel but would also have some sort of label that said 'rich in B_{12}' or 'vegetarian source of B_{12}'," says Michael Cohen, president of Lightlife Food, a Greenfield, Massachusetts, company that's one of the nation's largest producers of tempeh. "It was a major marketing point for tempeh manufacturers and one we had to let go of because we really couldn't stand behind it."

The new view of tempeh is due in part to better testing. Tests that originally determined that B_{12} was in tempeh have been found to be detecting other substances. It may also be the case that the industry's improved hygienic techniques have destroyed the B_{12}-carrying bacteria that were once in these foods. "If vegetables do contain B_{12}, that's an indirect way of saying they're contaminated with helpful bacteria," says Robert H. Allen, M.D., of the University of Colorado Health Sciences Center. "When vegetarians from India moved to England . . . B_{12} problems increased because the food was less contaminated with bacteria."

So, experts say, strict vegetarians should take a B_{12} supplement, which can be in pill form, since presumably they would have no trouble absorbing the vitamin.

boost or any other benefit if you don't have a deficiency. It's also not a one-time cure; if you need extra B$_{12}$ now, you're going to need it for the rest of your life. So there's no point in getting B$_{12}$ injections without being tested for deficiency. "Otherwise, at best, you're wasting your money," says Dr. Herbert.

Getting Your B$_{12}$

For all the hoopla over B$_{12}$, you need surprisingly little of it—one ten-millionth of an ounce daily. In fact, it's pretty hard not to get enough B$_{12}$ in your diet. (Remember, B$_{12}$ deficiency is usually due to stomach problems that prevent the vitamin from being absorbed.)

B$_{12}$ is found only in animal products, such as meats (particularly liver), eggs, and milk. "If it swims, flies, or runs, it has B$_{12}$," says Dr. Herbert. Only strict vegetarians (and especially their newborn offspring) need be concerned about B$_{12}$ deficiency through diet. But even for vegetarians, it takes a long time—perhaps ten years or more—to become deficient, because the body stores B$_{12}$ in abundance.

PART VI:
BETTER WAYS TO BEAT
EVERYDAY HEALTH PROBLEMS

Flash Reports

COMPARISON SHOPPING
FOR DENTAL FILLINGS

These days, dental fillings come in silver, gold, or resin materials. With these choices comes the obvious question: Which is best?

Silver amalgam fillings, actually a mix of silver, mercury, copper, and tin, are still the most common fillings. The American Dental Association says such fillings are safe and serviceable. They're also the most economical choice for fillings. But they're not always the best.

In some cases, gold is better. Why? Gold expands and contracts more like natural tooth enamel. So teeth filled with gold are less likely to crack than those filled with silver. Also, silver fillings may need to be replaced as often as every five years; gold may last as long as you do. Unfortunately, you pay for what you get. Gold fillings cost four times more than silver.

Before you decide between the silver and gold, consider too the composite resin fillings, newcomers that can match your natural teeth in color. Because resin fillings adhere to a tooth's surface, they require less drilling than metal fillings. And less drilling means less chance of breakage in later years. Also, better adhesion makes resin the preferred material for filling shallow surface cavities. Another advantage: They insulate sensitive teeth from extreme temperatures, while metal fillings conduct cold and heat, aggravating sensitive teeth. On the cost ledger, resins run just a little more than silver—and may last just as long.

SAFEGUARD
YOUR EYES' HEALTH

If you wear contact lenses, keep an eye out for *Acanthamoeba* keratitis, an infection caused by microorganisms that can lurk in nonsterile water. This rare but painful and potentially blinding disease is on the rise, yet doctors say proper prevention could all but eliminate it.

What makes *Acanthamoeba* keratitis so dangerous is that it's often not detected in its early stages. Its symptoms— eye pain, irritation, blurred vision, and sensitivity to light—are similar to those of many other eye problems. Positive diagnosis can be made only with a special laboratory technique that identifies the parasite. In addition, the disease is often difficult to treat, sometimes requiring cornea transplants.

Most cases are associated with using homemade saline solutions of distilled water and salt tablets to clean and store contact lenses. Economical, yes. Safe, no. Sterilizing the saline solution at home is difficult or impossible for most people.

Experts offer the following advice for reducing the risk of the disease. Use one of two proper sterilizing techniques: a hydrogen peroxide system or heat disinfection with commercial, sterile saline. Never wear contacts longer than your ophthalmologist recommends. If you're a soft-lens wearer, have your lenses replaced regularly. Consider wearing glasses instead of contacts when you're exposed to dust, dirt, or water, where the parasite may live. And always have any problem with your eyes or lenses checked immediately.

KEEPING CAVITIES OUT

Don't be surprised if you've never heard of dental sealants—safe, plastic coatings that your dentist places on
children's back teeth during the cavity-prone years, keeping out decay-causing food and bacteria for as long as a
decade. In a 1985 national survey, only 18 percent of adults
knew about sealants, even though the Surgeon General
and prestigious dental groups supported this form of tooth
protection.

Many dentists still don't use sealants. Possible reasons:
The first sealants, which appeared in 1971, weren't as good
as today's; older dentists may not have learned how to
apply them; a few practitioners think it's better to treat
cavities than prevent them; and some insurance companies
don't reimburse for the procedure.

Sealants, nevertheless, are widely available and are considered smart preventives for children, especially those
aged 6 to 14. To find a dentist who applies the coatings,
call your local dental society or a nearby dental school, or
ask your friends with children about their dentists.

CHAPTER 28

Ten
Medicine-Chest Musts

*These essential healers are the backbone of your personal
first-aid stash.*

There's an art to stocking a medicine chest. While you
might be tempted to keep something on hand for every
complaint known to man or woman, a cabinet over-
crowded with out-of-date or seldom-used medications is

not in your best interest. Stick to the essentials: a thermometer, tweezers, and a first-aid kit—plus a carefully chosen collection of "healers and helpers" to get you through those everyday aches, pains, and abrasions.

Choose products that offer maximum relief with minimum side effects. And to save money and reduce clutter, look to items that have a variety of uses—we call them *universal* healers. Don't stock up with multisymptom cold concoctions, however. According to Arthur H. Kibbe, Ph.D., director of scientific affairs for the American Pharmaceutical Association, it's best to tailor treatment to your specific cold complaints—something you can't do until you're in the throes of a full-blown viral attack.

Here, now, are ten over-the-counter essentials to keep on hand for other common assaults and minor body malfunctions. If a condition persists or recurs chronically, you should consult your doctor.

Petrolatum

Also known as petroleum jelly, this universal healer is many dermatologists' number one pick. Use it to protect and help heal dry, chafed, chapped, or wind-burned skin—from lips to elbows to heels. "Dry skin is a very common problem. It can become itchy, flaky, inflamed, and if left untreated, develop painful cracks and fissures, opening the door for infection," says Bernett Johnson, M.D., vice chairman of the Department of Dermatology at the University of Pennsylvania School of Medicine. Petrolatum works by providing a physical barrier to evaporation. Apply it to damp skin after a bath, Dr. Johnson recommends.

Unfortunately, the chief characteristic that makes petrolatum so useful—its greasiness—also makes it messy to use. As an alternative, you may want to use a moisturizer, especially during the day.

Petrolatum is also useful for diaper rash, for hemorrhoids, and to protect and soothe minor burns or sunburned skin. If your skin chafes when you walk or run, try applying some petrolatum to the strategic point on your skin before exercise.

Antacids

Heartburn, upset stomach, ulcers, indigestion, gastritis: Antacids can soothe them all! A common cause of stomach upset is too much acid, or stomach acid spilling over where it doesn't belong. In heartburn, for example, stomach acid backs up into the esophagus, causing that characteristic burning sensation that many people know all too well. Antacids neutralize the acid, relieving the discomfort.

"The most commonly used and effective antacids are the aluminum and magnesium hydroxide compounds," says Samuel Klein, M.D., assistant professor in the Division of Gastroenterology at the University of Texas Medical Branch.

Aspirin

Few healers can beat the universal appeal of aspirin. Everyone knows that aspirin is a potent pain reliever for headaches, toothaches, and menstrual cramps. But because it also reduces inflammation, aspirin is especially soothing for arthritis and injuries like strains and sprains. In a study at the University of Alabama, 20 women who were given two aspirin four times a day had less soreness and a greater range of motion two days after performing some unusual arm exercises than volunteers who didn't take aspirin. The researchers speculate that aspirin's anti inflammatory effect was responsible for the reduction in "delayed muscle soreness." Aspirin can also help reduce a fever—good news for an achy, feverish flu sufferer!

Note: Children or teenagers with the flu or chicken pox should avoid aspirin because of a possible link with Reye's syndrome.

If aspirin upsets your stomach, or if you are allergic to it, acetaminophen is a good substitute. Acetaminophen also relieves pain and fever, but not inflammation. Ibuprofen relieves pain, inflammation, and fever. Some people prefer it to aspirin, especially for menstrual cramps. Ultimately, however, your choice of pain reliever may simply come down to whatever works best for you. Just be aware that if you are allergic to aspirin, ibuprofen is generally off-limits, too.

Athlete's-Foot Powder

The fungus that causes athlete's foot runs rampant on all kinds of feet—not just those belonging to jocks. In fact, as many as 50 percent of people test positive for the infection at one time or another, according to Norman Klombers, D.P.M., executive director of the American Podiatric Medical Association. The fungus is so widespread that you can come in contact with it even if you never set foot on a locker-room floor. And, once exposed, most people do an excellent job of growing the fungus. "Every day we put our feet inside a pair of socks inside a pair of shoes. That dark, warm, moist environment is a perfect incubator for athlete's-foot fungus," says Dr. Klombers.

Daily care becomes essential to kill the fungus and prevent a serious outbreak. After a shower, be sure to dry your feet well, especially between the toes. Then apply a very light dusting of athlete's-foot powder before dressing. And take note, more is *not* better; if you use too much powder, you'll clog the pores, and moisture will accumulate—the very thing you're trying to avoid.

Antibiotic Ointment

These ointments use a shotgun approach to prevent infection in cuts and scrapes: They contain two or three different antibiotics, each effective against a different range of bacteria, to make sure that nothing grows in a wound except skin.

And, according to a study, they're preferable to most traditional antiseptics. Researchers at the University of Pennsylvania compared the effectiveness of triple-antibiotic ointment with that of double-antibiotic ointment and with that of a wide assortment of first-aid creams and antiseptic sprays and lotions. Old standbys, such as Mercurochrome, Merthiolate, hydrogen peroxide, and tincture of iodine, were also put to the test. Wounds treated with triple-antibiotic and double-antibiotic ointment healed in about 9.2 and 8.8 days—faster and better than those treated with anything else. By comparison, wounds treated with hydrogen peroxide healed in 14.3 days, and iodine-treated cuts healed in 15.7 days. Interestingly, wounds receiving no treatment at all healed in 13.2 days, beating out some of the nonantibiotic preparations.

Why did the antiseptics fare so poorly compared with the antibiotic ointments?

"Antiseptics that hurt when you apply them to a wound do so because they're doing damage—actually injuring tissue," says Dr. Kibbe. Also, according to Dr. Johnson, some studies suggest that keeping a wound moist aids healing because the new cells can move into place more quickly. That may be another reason that the ointments were superior. The ingredients to look for are neomycin, polymyxin B, and bacitracin.

Just for the record, be sure to clean the wound with soap and water before applying the ointment. Cover with a bandage, if necessary. And, of course, if a cut is deep or too large to be closed with an adhesive bandage, seek medical help as soon as possible.

Salt

What's this doing in the medicine chest rather than the pantry? Lots. Warm salt water is one of the most useful and natural healers around. Gargle with it to soothe a sore throat and kill germs. (The higher concentration of salt kills germs by sucking them dry, a process that works by osmotic pressure.) You can also use warm salt water as a mouthwash to firm up gum tissue or to treat a mouth injury, as nose drops to relieve congestion when you have a cold, or as an eyewash to treat eye inflammation.

To make an eyewash, use ½ teaspoon of salt in an eight-ounce glass of distilled warm water. Discard the leftover saline solution.

You can even use salt water as a first line of defense to fend off vaginitis, says Gideon G. Panter, M.D., assistant professor of obstetrics and gynecology at Cornell University Medical College. "Bathing in a tub of warm water in which ½ cup of salt has been dissolved helps restore the normal pH and ecology of the vagina," he says. "Do this several nights in a row at the first sign of abnormal discharge or itching, and nine times out of ten you'll save yourself a trip to the doctor."

Hydrocortisone Cream

Available in low-dose over-the-counter preparations, hydrocortisone cream can relieve the itch and swelling of hemorrhoids. But it is most commonly used to soothe minor skin irritations—mild cases of contact dermatitis, insect bites, poison ivy or oak, and small patches of sunburn. Dab a little on, rub it in lightly, and leave the area unbandaged. "Heavy applications are unnecessary, since the drug will not diffuse from the top of a thick layer of cream," says Dr. Kibbe. "And don't use hydrocortisone on large areas or on broken skin without consulting a doctor."

Antidiarrheal

Most cases of simple diarrhea go away with or without treatment. All you have to do is hang in for about 24 hours. But why suffer?! A diarrhea remedy can help soothe your gastrointestinal tract, stop the cramping, and ease the discomfort. Products containing the combination of kaolin and pectin are a good choice and are very safe, says Dr. Klein. But again, it comes down to personal preference; you may find that other products work best for you.

Note: You should check with your doctor before using antidiarrhea medication if you have a fever or blood in your stool. And seek medical help if the diarrhea lasts more than 72 hours.

Ice Pack

Although this is technically not found in the medicine chest, it is a must in every home, especially for active people.

Cold, or cryotherapy, is an excellent first-aid treatment for acute injuries, such as muscle strains, sprains, and bruises. It helps stop internal bleeding from injured blood vessels by causing them to constrict. The less blood that collects around the injury, the shorter the healing time. Cold also reduces pain, swelling, and muscle spasm.

Choose any kind of ice pack that conforms to the contours of your body. A gel pack that's kept in the freezer is fine. So is a good old-fashioned rubberized ice bag. In a pinch, you can even use a bag of frozen peas. Just don't rest it directly on your skin—wrap it in a towel.

Apply the ice pack to your injury for 15 minutes, let the area warm for 15 minutes, then reapply the ice pack. You can repeat this for up to several hours.

You can even prevent pain by massaging an injury with ice before exercising.

Applying an ice pack can also alleviate bursitis and reduce headache pain in some people, and ice can even take the itch out of insect bites and the sting out of minor burns.

Laxative

The best treatment for constipation is prevention—eating a high-fiber diet, drinking plenty of water, and getting regular exercise. But occasionally, even the best of us get blocked up and need help. So for those times, it's essential to have a laxative on hand. Just remember: The milder the product, the better, says Dr. Kibbe. Bulk-forming laxatives, especially those containing psyllium seeds, are the best choice.

Avoid stimulant-type laxatives. They can lead to laxative dependence, a condition that can result in permanent damage to your colon. Consult a pharmacist or physician for help in choosing the product that's safest for you.

CHAPTER 29
Triumph Over Back Pain

This intensive, nonsurgical back clinic requires eight hours a day of rehabbing.

Michael Foley knew exactly how he'd hurt his back. The 27-year-old fireman slipped in oil on the station house floor and landed hard on his butt. He'd been in and out of the hospital for eight months, using a wheelchair and taking heavy-duty painkillers. But that's all behind him now. Today, just a few weeks after enrolling in a very special back rehabilitation program, Michael is ready to return to work. To prove it, he staged a test run—in fire-fighting fashion—from the hospital roof. Using ropes, he hauled his counselor down the side of the five-story building.

An unusual case? Not at the University of Miami's Comprehensive Pain and Rehabilitation Center. Here, people with chronic back pain—who've spent more time in bed than out, tried doctor after doctor to no avail, lost jobs and spouses as a result, and worst of all, been told to learn to live with their pain—triumph over seemingly impossible odds. Most return home with a significant reduction in pain and the skills necessary to get on with their lives, says founding director Hubert Rosomoff, M.D. And many, like Michael Foley, graduate from the four-week program virtually pain free and functional—without surgery. (For more information on the University of Miami's Comprehensive Pain and Rehabilitation Center, write the center at 600 Alton Road, Miami Beach, FL 33139. Or to locate a physiatrist in your area, contact the Association of Academic Physiatrists, 8000 Five Mile Road, Suite 340, Cincinnati, OH 45230, or call (513) 232-8833.)

Exercising Your Alternatives

Why does this program succeed where others fail? Much of the credit goes to Dr. Rosomoff. A well-known neurosurgeon, he found that many of his back patients on a presurgery exercise program improved so much they didn't need an operation. So he set aside his scalpel and developed an exercise regimen that's become the core of the rehabilitation program. The results are remarkable; even patients who'd been warned that exercise could leave them crippled have benefited.

Most back pain, he contends, is the result of weakened muscles. Back muscles need to be strong and flexible. Otherwise, even small movements can throw them into painful spasms. Unfortunately, with age, muscles stiffen unless they're stretched and worked. And torn or pulled muscles tighten as they mend, especially with too much rest.

This weakness in the musculature of the back has a name: It's called myofascial syndrome. *Myofascial* refers to the muscles, ligaments, and connective tissue that support the vertebrae of the spine and wrap around the hips, buttocks, and stomach. This, Dr. Rosomoff believes, is the source of more than 90 percent of all back pain.

Slipped disks or pinched nerves (which, incidentally, cause numbness and tingling, not pain) can result from muscle weakness, too, he explains. Many people with these problems—as well as those with spinal misalignment, degenerative disk disease, or arthritis—can benefit from a well-designed back-strengthening exercise program. "Too often, we see people who've had unnecessary surgery," Dr. Rosomoff notes. "They still hurt, and now they have an additional problem—scar tissue from the incision, which makes their backs even stiffer."

Team Healing

At the University of Miami's Comprehensive Pain and Rehabilitation Center, physical-medicine specialists, psychologists, occupational therapists, vocational counselors, and others team up to get patients back on track, without surgery. It's the only back clinic in America with ergonomists on staff. (Ergonomists are industrial engineers who specialize in people's anatomical relationship to their work environment.)

The doctors who oversee a patient's total care are physiatrists (physicians who specialize in physical medicine and rehabilitation). They have a strong background in muscle/ skeleton structure and the nervous system and are knowledgeable about nonsurgical treatments. They are also experts in evaluating many types of back pain.

The Power of the Participants

Of course, for all the expertise the staff offers, the real key to the success of this program is what the patients bring to it: determination and hard work. As an older woman with spinal arthritis confided, "When my doctor told me I had to live with my pain, I thought to myself, 'I can't live with it.' That's when I made up my mind to come to the center."

It's no coincidence that among the reading material in the center's conference room is the children's classic *The Little Engine That Could*. It's a story about a tiny but determined steam engine that pulls a long train up a steep hill. That book has personal significance for chronic back pain patients whose lives have become uphill battles.

To ensure that program participants don't quit halfway up the hill, the center requires patients to sign a written agreement to work eight hours a day on back rehabbing. They also agree, in writing, to try to meet specific work and personal goals.

"Personal goals are powerful motivators," says Renee Steele Rosomoff, the center's program director. One patient, a UPS delivery man, said he needed to drive a truck for two hours without stopping, lift up to 80 pounds over his head 100 times a day, and walk half a mile without pain. Another, a Vietnam vet, was determined to leave the clinic on his beloved motorcycle—no small feat, considering he arrived in a wheelchair! Both met their goals.

A Taste of the Offerings

What's it like to participate in the program at this unique back-saving center? Starting on day one, you'll join other patients in a large activity room filled with floor mats, mirrors, weight-lifting equipment, and therapy tables. (Off this room is a special refuge—a soothing whirlpool, plus a private therapy room.) Here, your back will feel like the fleshy equivalent of a rusty hinge; you'll need to loosen it up to get it moving again (it may creak just as much!).

You'll lie on a padded table for a deep muscle massage. The therapist will slowly turn your head to the left, then right, as she strokes the muscles from your shoulders to the base of your head. She'll knead your buttocks and hamstrings (sometimes using her elbow!). Then you'll roll over onto your back for a knees-to-chest stretch. Stretching can hurt at first, so the therapist rubs ice in small circles over the sore spots.

If you're especially stiff, you may benefit from a session on the gravity-traction, or auto-traction, table. Strapped to the table in a kind of harness, you're raised vertically, head up. This allows the weight of your lower body to gently pull at your spine. Some people find this process painful at first, as tight muscles give way. Gradually, it becomes relaxing—so much so, you'll soon feel like reading a novel during this treatment.

But don't get too relaxed; you've got to get on with your stretching exercises. A physical therapist will show you the proper way to stretch the muscles around your tail-bone, hips, thighs, shoulders, and neck. He emphasizes the importance of using slow, steady motions and holding each pose at full range of motion for six seconds. Remember that; you're expected to repeat the stretching exercises on your own, several times a day.

Another reminder: Don't stop stretching because your muscles ache. They will initially. Work through the stiffness. The dull ache associated with exercise should start to subside by the third week. (If you experience swelling, bruises, or sharp pain, however, stop immediately. These symptoms indicate pulled or torn muscles.)

Back-Saving Muscle Building

You also will need to strengthen the same muscles you're stretching—and a few more besides (see "Best Back Strengtheners"). Your abdominal muscles (which, believe it or not, provide your back's main support) definitely need firming up. So do the muscles on the front of your arms (biceps) and thighs (quadriceps).

Strong biceps and quadriceps can save your back when it comes to lifting heavy packages. If you hunch over to scoop up a bag of groceries, you're making your upper

Best Back Strengtheners

Follow these exercises to strengthen your back, pelvic, and abdominal muscles.

Pelvic tilt. Stand with your back and shoulders against a wall, your feet at shoulder width and your heels about eight inches from the wall. Bend your knees slightly, then tighten your buttocks and pull in your stomach. Try to make the small of your back touch the wall. Hold for a count of six. Relax upward, then repeat. Once you've got the hang of it, do it without the wall! This simple stance instantly relieves lower back strain when lifting and standing.

Curls. Lie on your back and bend both knees. Begin to exhale slowly while lifting first your head, then your shoulders, off the mat. With your arms outstretched, hold for six seconds.

Side-to-side sit-ups. Lie on your back with knees bent and feet on the floor. Touch your chin to your chest, stretch your arms forward, and slowly curl up, reaching toward the right (or left) knee. Hold for six seconds.

"Cat" pose. Get on your hands and knees, with lower back relaxed. Drop your head, pull in your stomach muscles, and make your back as rounded and high as possible. Hold for six seconds.

Butt tucks. Lie on your back, knees bent and feet flat. Push down and lift your buttocks off the floor. Your shoulders should remain on the mat. Hold five seconds, then slowly return to the floor.

back do the biceps' work. Rather, extend your arms to bring the bag up to your chest. Likewise, you need to flex your knees, tuck in your stomach, and bend at the hips to lift objects without straining your lower back. For that stance, you need strong "quads." Bicycling is a great quad builder. That's why you're required to put in a respectable number of miles each day on a stationary bike.

The Art of Relaxation

Within a few days of arrival, you'll be hooked up to an electromyographic biofeedback machine. This device measures electrical activity in muscle groups and projects it as a bar graph on a TV screen or as beeps on a portable receiver. It's used to monitor posture, movements, and muscle relaxation.

Like a constantly correcting teacher, biofeedback can be annoying at first, as Celia Stern discovered. Her spinal arthritis had left her hunched over and so stiff that even grocery shopping was torture. She'd seen how straightening up, keeping her shoulders down and her neck erect but relaxed stilled the machine's beeper. That meant she was putting minimum stress on her upper back muscles. The trick, though, was to keep the infernal thing quiet even while she lifted and moved a five-pound weight from a kitchen counter to a grocery cart! With guidance from a staff member, she tried, again and again, to hold the correct postures as she moved. After numerous attempts, she was finally able to do so, although she'd still need to practice, practice, practice.

Biofeedback can help you learn to relax tense muscles, too. If your shoulders are tense, for instance, a therapist attaches biofeedback sensors to your stiff muscles. In some cases, she can help you develop an image or sensation that lets you relax. For example, she may instruct you to visualize your shoulders bathed in warm sunlight. "Let your arms hang at your sides, imagining them heavier and heavier," she continues. "Feel your shoulders drop with each deep exhalation." In case you can't recognize a state of relaxation, the machine lets you know when you've achieved it.

The Workplace Analysts

Most people who enroll in this program expect to return full-time to their previous jobs. To make sure they do, the staff re-creates each person's work environment and analyzes it for its back-stressing potential. You'll need to supply photographs and measurements of your workplace.

The staff goes to great lengths to duplicate it. They have brought in delivery trucks, propane gas tanks, even railroad switches for people to practice their new "work smart" postures. Sometimes the staff ergonomist suggests simple changes in the workplace; other times, people are shown how best to work around existing conditions.

Almost every job has its pitfalls. Paper shuffling can be just as hard on your back as ditch digging, as Ruth Ryals, an insurance specialist for a large company, knows. Her back pain made it impossible for her to sit at her desk for prolonged periods.

In the ergonomics lab, hooked up to a biofeedback machine at her simulated workplace, she sees exactly what movements stress her back. Dangling her feet from a too-high chair sends the biofeedback machine into a frenzy of beeps. Putting her feet up on a low stool completely quiets it. Reaching over her desk for a heavy file sets it off again. Standing up and sliding the file forward causes only an occasional beep. Twisting to look over her shoulder to read a calendar creates a crescendo of electronic noise. The ergonomist suggests she post a second calendar on the opposite side of her desk.

Little Things Add Up

There's no magic bullet to stop back pain. But at this rehabilitation center, you learn there are tons of little things that work just fine. Graduates from the program are expected to continue to exercise, walk, or bike at least half an hour twice a day, to continue to lose weight if necessary, to think before they lift, to ask for help if they need it, and to throttle back, but only for a day or two, when flare-ups occur.

"I know exactly what I need to do to keep my back in shape," says Michael Foley. "Over time, those habits have become automatic."

CHAPTER 30

50 Facts and Tips to Help Tame Allergies

Learn how drinking ice water can cure postnasal drip, why chronic hives are really bug bites, and more.

"The practice of allergy has become overly complicated and complex," says Ralph Bookman, M.D. "It's essentially a very simple subject, and unfortunately, some of its most effective treatments have been all but forgotten."

An old-school scholar, Dr. Bookman is an associate clinical professor at the University of Southern California School of Medicine and a member of the advisory council of the National Institute of Allergy and Infectious Diseases. Still, he finds time to make his own allergy extracts and dispense highly opinionated advice to patients—including former president Ronald Reagan—four days a week.

Here, then, are dozens of his treatments, tips, explanations, and opinions culled from a series of interviews and from Dr. Bookman's excellent book, *The Dimensions of Clinical Allergy.*

1. **Positive reactions are not positive proof.** The first thing that happens when an allergic person inhales, ingests, or physically contacts an allergen is that he or she becomes sensitized to it. All that means is that the body now recognizes that substance distinctly—it doesn't mean that exposure is going to cause them to experience symptoms.

    But it will cause them to react to that substance when

skin tested. These positive reactions tend to convince people that they're allergic to many more things than they really are.

2. **Thresholds.** Even when people are allergic to a substance, there is a certain level of exposure they can tolerate before symptoms appear. Exceed that threshold, and up pop the symptoms.

   Most people already understand that the same amount of pollen can bother one allergic person and not another. What they often fail to understand is that thresholds can also vary widely in the same person over a period of time.

3. **Where's your "dial" set today?** Generally these changes occur gradually during a person's lifetime. Without changing a thing around them, some people's sensitivities to one substance can all but vanish, while other allergies reappear after years of absence.

   Dr. Bookman likes to say that the "dial setting" of their allergic responsiveness has changed. Most times, this occurs slowly and subtly, but some events can cause immediate changes in a person's dial setting.

4. **Shots and sickness work the same.** Allergy injections don't get rid of your allergy to a substance—they raise your threshold, so that you can tolerate more of the substance before you experience allergy symptoms.

   But a virus has almost the same effect, temporarily. It's not unusual to see allergic skin lesions clear or respiratory symptoms disappear during a virus attack. Surgery or other major trauma, such as breaking a bone, almost invariably shuts down allergy symptoms as well.

5. **Allergy symptoms: There are only three.** All allergic symptoms are a combination of three basic effects. Nothing more. There is edema (swelling), particularly of the skin and mucus membrane. There is an increase in the secretion of mucus, especially in the respiratory tract. And, less important, there is spasm of smooth muscle where smooth muscle exists.

6. **A little swelling can make a big impact.** Several areas adjacent to the respiratory tract have one thing in common: They're so small that very little edema is necessary

to obstruct them. These include the middle ear and the olfactory recess, which controls our sense of smell.

When episodes of sinus pain, middle-ear problems, and loss of sense of smell occur, look to allergy as the cause.

7. **Alcohol augments allergies.** Alcohol is not an allergen. But it does act to congest the nasal passages. In someone with allergic rhinitis (a runny, stuffed-up, allergic nose), it adds to the edema already present due to allergies.

   Some people with allergies are unable to drink at all because of the intense nasal congestion that alcohol produces. Dr. Booker sometimes wonders if a lot of hangovers aren't the result of alcohol-induced sinus blockage.

8. **Smoke is not an allergen.** A lot of people claim to be allergic to tobacco smoke, but the large molecules necessary for an allergic reaction can't survive the burning heat of a cigarette.

   There are cases of true tobacco allergy, but they always involve physical contact with the raw leaf. Cigarette smoke can make you cough, sneeze, and wheeze, but it's not an allergy, and allergy treatments won't prevent it or clear it up.

9. **Irritants, not allergens.** A large number of nonprotein substances, such as tissues, paper dust, paint fumes, perfume, and newsprint, are erroneously called allergens. They do produce symptoms in many people, but it's because they're irritating, not because they're allergens.

10. **Could "chronic hives" be bug bites?** Dr. Booker finds it odd that so many pediatricians and dermatologists report seeing patients with chronic hives when he has never encountered such a person. He says that he has seen the persistent itchy little bumps these physicians describe, but they are invariably the result of insect bites.

    Their appearance on the legs is a strong clue that the culprit is fleas. These little creatures are tenaciously hard to eliminate from the home and rarely jump higher than 18 inches to bite their prey.

11. **Not all seasonal allergies are pollen.** Steer manure, a popular lawn fertilizer, contains copious amounts of cattle dander, which is a very potent allergen. Because it's generally applied in the spring or fall, people often mistake the seasonal symptoms as an allergy to pollens.

12. **Pups no problem.** Very young animals have no old skin to shed and therefore have no dander. It usually takes a couple of months before such pets produce their allergen, which may explain why some people "suddenly" become allergic to a dog or cat they got as a pup or kitten.

13. **Pet myths miss the point.** Legend has it that poodles don't cause allergy problems. The fact is that they may have less dander to give off because they are the breed that is washed and groomed most frequently.

    Also, chihuahuas are thought to be "safe" pets because they are hairless. But hair is actually not the problem! It probably just takes a long time for such a small dog to give off sufficient quantities of dander to put a person over their allergic threshold.

14. **Pets—or pollen?** Cats and dogs that are allowed to roam freely through their environments often play in grassy and weed-strewn areas, where they can pick up quite a bit of pollen in their pelts.

    Some people who think they're allergic to pets are actually reacting to the pet-borne pollen and not to the pets.

15. **Too much dander and nothing works!** The amount of dander deposited on a home's rugs and furniture by a pet is usually far greater than allergy injections can ever hope to overcome.

    The shots won't really help until the pets are moved outdoors and the dander has been thoroughly cleaned out of all the rugs and furniture.

16. **Goat hair? In the White House?** Most people have a lot more animal dander in their environment than they realize. If they have a true Oriental rug, for instance, then it is certainly loaded with sheep, goat, and camel dander.

    President Reagan always said he felt much better at

Camp David than at the White House, and that's not surprising to Dr. Booker. The White House is full of antique furniture stuffed with animal hair. When someone plops down in one of those old chairs or couches, a ton of dander comes blowing into the room.

Camp David has all new furniture. And new furniture isn't filled with dander.

17. **Wool worries.** Good-quality domestic wool is processed to be dander free; it is not allergenic. However, it is irritating to many people—and not just those with allergies.

Wool from Third World countries is not treated after it's taken from the animal. This kind of wool can contain a lot of dander and cause serious allergy problems.

18. **Allergy relief begins in the bedroom.** Since we spend half our lives in the bedroom, this is the area where controls will be the most effective.

Of course the living room contains allergens! But the short amount of time that we spend there generally doesn't justify the expense and inconvenience necessary to remedy its faults.

Time and energy spent in allergy-proofing the bedroom, however, will be well returned in reduced symptoms.

19. **Pillow power.** All pillows must be synthetic. Dr. Booker has found Dacron to be the most comfortable substitute for feather pillows.

Forget allergy encasings. They don't work well on pillows unless the zipper is airtight, and that makes the pillow like a balloon, since the air can't escape.

20. **Pass on pillows for headache relief.** Of 75 headache patients Dr. Booker tested, all but a very few were found to be strongly allergic to environmental (indoor) allergens.

A few ended their headaches with simple environmental controls, such as removal of a down comforter, feather pillows, or a pet. One patient's head pain was relieved by the removal of a bedroom chair found to contain goat hair.

21. **Blanket protection.** Wool blankets are not only irritating, they're notorious dust collectors. Turn off the lights

in the bedroom, shine a flashlight across the bed, and slap down on the blanket with your free hand. You'll probably see a very convincing cloud of dust.

Synthetic blankets should be used, since they don't collect dust as readily. Down comforters, of course, must be removed.

22. **Down or dog, it's still all dander.** In all reactions to animals, only the dander is significant. The hairs and feathers have no allergic potential themselves but are always contaminated by dander, which is nothing more than old skin scales.

   Each feather, if examined carefully, shows the presence of dried dander at its base. This dander remains despite commercial cleaning, which is why down can be highly allergenic even when old.

23. **Fun fur's no fun.** Rabbit, when used as a "fun fur" or in an angora sweater, can be a source of allergy symptoms because the fur is too delicate to withstand the kind of cleaning that would get all the dander out. Most other costume furs are dander free, but contact-allergy symptoms sometimes develop from the lacquer used to color the fur.

24. **Is all asthma allergic?** Almost everyone in the medical community looks at bronchial asthma and allergic rhinitis (hay fever) as separate and distinct entities. Dr. Booker looks at them both as manifestations of respiratory allergy.

   After all, the same mucous membrane lines the respiratory tract from top to bottom, and the changes that occur in the nose and sinus in allergy are virtually identical to the changes that occur in the bronchial tree during an asthma attack.

   If physicians look at the similarities of the conditions instead of their differences, Dr. Booker theorizes, they can better treat the patient as a whole.

25. **Asthma? See an allergist!** Asthmatics treated by a good allergist are hospitalized much less frequently than those under the care of other types of physicians. That's because all asthma is allergic. If more physicians realized this, asthma would be treated much more efficiently in this country, Dr. Booker says.

26. **Moderate asthma is the worst.** It's the person with low-grade, moderate asthma who benefits the most from competent medical help. These people suffer constant low-level wheezing and shortness of breath that makes them irritable, miserable, and tired all the time. Dr. Booker believes that the additional muscular effort each breath takes for these people is a very common cause of fatigue.

27. **"Frequent colds" are frequently allergies.** Physicians' offices are filled with patients complaining of frequent colds. It is unfortunate that these people's symptoms aren't recognized for what they are: allergic rhinitis that would respond well to specific allergy care.

    Dr. Booker says that he has had patients tell him that they only have two colds a year. But when the patients are questioned, he finds out that the first "cold" tends to last as long as the spring pollen season, while the second coincides perfectly with the fall pollen season!

28. **Cold or allergy?** A cold is an upper respiratory infection, and it displays the typical symptoms of infection: low-grade fever, purulent nasal discharge, and a general malaise that lasts from three to five days. It also has a tendency to be transmitted from one family member to another.

    Continuous episodes of sneezing, with a watery nasal discharge, nasal obstruction, and head congestion, accompanied by a sense of fatigue that lingers for weeks or longer, can be reasonably assumed to be allergic.

29. **All septums are deviated!** No biological entity has a body part that is ruler straight; therefore no one has a perfectly straight septum! They all deviate from the vertical to some degree. The only effect of a deviated septum is to make one nasal passage larger and the other smaller. There is no real effect on total air flow.

    When swelling occurs, the smaller one quite naturally blocks before the larger one, but the final effect on air flow is the same as if both sides were equal.

30. **Leave it bent.** In most cases, Dr. Booker sees little reason to straighten a septum, and the temporary im-

provement you see after straightening is the same allergy-deadening effect you can expect from any surgery. The swelling and obstruction generally return in a few weeks, after your body recovers from the trauma of the surgery.

31. **That stuck-in-the-throat feeling.** Some people with postnasal drip develop swelling in an area of the throat called the uvula. Because this area has little sensory discrimination, the swelling feels as if there's mucus trapped there that can't be dislodged. Drinking ice water can reduce the swelling and eliminate that feeling of trapped mucus.

32. **Allergic hoarseness.** Many people with allergies often experience a painless hoarseness. Look down their throat and you'll find swelling and pallor rather than the red, "angry," painful inflammation caused by overuse. Using an epinephrine inhaler (like Primatene Mist) can eliminate the edema that's causing the problem.

    People who use their voices professionally—singers, actors, and announcers—often experience gratifying results when they use such an inhaler before speaking or singing. But it won't help if the problem is nonallergic and just due to overuse.

33. **Antihistamine advice.** If there were one or two reliable antihistamines that worked for everyone, the rest would evaporate and be forgotten. But that, of course, is not the case—their effectiveness and side effects are different in everyone.

    Patients should be given small starter packs so they can find the antihistamine that works best for them. They should also avoid driving until they are certain of how drowsy a specific antihistamine makes them.

    Some produce such a powerful sedation that they may help an allergic patient not so much by controlling their symptoms but simply by helping them get a good night's sleep!

34. **And a warning. . . .** Antihistamines function well in allergy partly because of their drying effect. But in asthma, the reverse—hydration—is necessary for the control of symptoms. Therefore, antihistamines

should never—repeat, never—be used when asthma symptoms are present. Dr. Booker prefers to use decongestants instead.

35. **Instant "allergic ear" relief!** Eustachian tube blockage can often be dramatically relieved with nasal sprays containing a strong decongestant, such as Neo-Synephrine (0.5 percent).

Tilt the head back and to one side, turn the spray bottle upside down, and get enough of the spray into the nasal passage so that you can actually taste some of it in the back of your throat. Then turn your head the other way and repeat, using the other nostril.

This technique is often dramatically effective at ending allergic ear problems, because it passes the decongestant directly over the entrance to the eustachian area located in the nasopharynx.

During plane flights, this should be done a half hour before a scheduled descent. For children, it should be done at the first sign of pain or discomfort, repeated in four hours, and repeated again if symptoms reappear. This often aborts painful episodes of otitis media.

36. **Tissues, not allergies, shred noses.** Red, raw, and chafed noses are thought by many to be a sign that allergies are present. They well may be, but the actual chafing damage is invariably due to the excessive use of paper tissues. All tissues are made of wood pulp and are extremely irritating.

Children often suffer heavily fissured, even infected, noses because mothers, in their zeal, insert the tissue into the nostril and twist vigorously. The condition is easily cured by using handkerchiefs or other cotton cloths and greasing the nostrils with petroleum jelly for protection.

37. **Wash your hands to prevent eye problems!** The skin of the fingers is notoriously resistant to allergy reactions, but the thin skin around the eyelids is extremely reactive. And the area of our body most often touched with the finger is the area around the eye. Washing hands immediately after handling pets, foods, and other problem substances can greatly reduce eye symptoms in allergic individuals.

38. **To stop the itch.** Two factors increase the itching in atopic dermatitis—exposure to the air and the presence of crusts and scales. The best treatment attends to both factors.

   Soaking in a tub filled with a handful of Epsom salts dissolved in comfortably warm bath water for 15 to 20 minutes several times a day removes crusts and scales. Ocean bathing can achieve the same result. Open lesions may sting a bit at first, but relief will come rapidly.

   After the bath, get dry and immediately apply boric acid ointment. In children, use petroleum jelly instead. It may seem messy, but it can greatly reduce itching by protecting the skin from exposure to the air.

   If the grease appears to inflame the skin further, use a water-soluble ointment, such as Aquaphor, instead.

39. **Allergic headache.** It is unfortunate that this common allergy symptom receives so little attention, since it responds to treatment more readily and more successfully than any other form of recurrent head pain.

   So-called cluster headaches that appear in the spring and fall are inevitably allergic responses to pollen. Indoor allergens are also a common headache cause.

40. **Migraine or allergy?** Both allergic and migraine headaches tend to appear early in life. Migraines, however, decrease in intensity as an individual gets older. Allergic headaches do not. And while migraines have a classic, distinctive appearance, allergic headache is characterized by the total absence of any specific pattern. Pain can occur anywhere in the head.

41. **Head pain? How's your nose?** There is a strong association between head pain and nasal congestion in allergic individuals. Many notice that their head pain is relieved at the same time as their congestion. Others notice considerable nasal discharge or a bubbling noise in the head as their headache improves, strongly suggesting that a sinus obstruction has been relieved.

42. **A positive mistake.** Sometimes a person will inadvertently receive an injection that is too strong during allergy therapy. The headache that quickly develops is the final diagnostic proof that their headaches are

allergic in origin and that the correct allergen is being used.

Many patients also note that their headaches return if they wait too long between injections.

43. **Pack your nose for head pain!** When head pain is definitely caused by blocked sinuses, there is a technique that brings quick relief. Saturate tufted cotton with a strong nasal decongestant, and using a twisting motion, pack as much into each nostril as you can tolerate, and leave it there for five minutes.

There's often dramatic relief of the pain, especially if you catch the headache early on. You can't do it more than once a day or it'll be too irritating, and you have to use tufted cotton in order to hold enough of the decongestant fluid. Cotton swabs won't do the job.

44. **Skin-test tips.** You can't predict the severity of a person's symptoms by their skin tests alone. Dr. Booker says he often sees large skin-test reactions in people with mild hay fever and small reactions in people who have severe allergy problems.

And not all people with allergic disease react when skin tested. Occasionally you'll see a person with a classic history of spring hay fever whose skin tests are negative. Such people generally respond well to injections of the pollens that are in the air when their symptoms are worst.

45. **Seniors can be skin tested.** Some doctors claim that elderly people don't react at all when skin tested. This is just not so. Older people tend not to flare (the redness that appears around a positive skin test), but the wheal (the actual hivelike welt that springs up when a test is positive) can be read if you look at it in oblique light and feel around to determine its size.

46. **Medical forms miss the mark.** Forms interfere with getting a good idea of a person's medical history for two reasons. First, they're created by doctors, using terms that doctors are familiar with but that many patients aren't. You get a lot of wrong answers simply because most people are going to misunderstand at least some of the words.

Second, all forms, no matter how carefully they are written, are extremely rigid in structure. This prevents a doctor from learning of unusual events that may be important for correct diagnosis and treatment.

47. **Doctors: Ask more questions!** A doctor should always ask patients what they mean when they say they "have a lot of colds" or when they complain of frequent infections. Are these infections, or just short-term worsening of allergic symptoms?

    People in cold climates often report lots of winter colds and infections. The real problem is that they're spending more time indoors, surrounded by indoor allergens.

48. **How to catch a mouth breather.** Doctors shouldn't bother asking people if they're mouth breathers, says Dr. Booker, because they're just going to say no. They should ask instead if the patient wakes up with a dry mouth or a sore throat in the morning—both are sure signs of mouth breathing! Hot drinks can relieve the problem quickly.

49. **"Women's mucus."** Women are often relieved to hear that it is not unusual for vaginal mucous discharge to increase when traditional allergy symptoms are most troublesome. This is especially true of seasonal allergy reactions, and it's a perfectly normal allergy symptom.

50. **Prescription: 40 winks!** The difficulty some of these people have in coping with life is due entirely to the fatigue their condition is causing. Nothing produces a more positive response in such people than allergy therapy that allows them to get a good night's sleep.

CHAPTER 31

Snore No More

A review of the best antisnoring treatments known, from the simple to the surgical.

Once and for all, let's bury these two myths about snoring: (1) There isn't a darn thing you can do about it if you're the snorer and very little (that's legal) if you're the snoree; and (2) snoring is just noise, either laughable or annoying, signifying nothing.

Science and medicine have given the lie to both of these. There are effective remedies for the nightly snorting and harrumphing. Snorers may be able to use self-care strategies to end the noise for good within a week in some cases, or in others, within a few months. Plus, there are doctors (called somnologists) who can successfully treat snoring and other sleep problems at various sleep disorder centers around the country. And we now know that not all snoring is just benign clatter. One type not only raises the roof but signals a potentially life-threatening—but correctable—condition.

Reasons for the Racket

About 45 percent of all adults snore occasionally; 25 percent are habitual snorers. And the vast majority of snorers are men. What causes all the noise? An obstruction in the airway, usually the tongue. Most often when a snorer relaxes during sleep, his tongue falls backward against the soft palate and other floppy tissues at the back of his throat. When he breathes, the stream of air that enters his throat causes the tongue and these tissues to vibrate against one another. And the farther his tongue drops back, the more vibrating, or snoring, occurs.

For about 30 percent of heavy snorers, the tongue drops back so far that it winds up getting sucked into the airway "like a moist cork," in the words of Chicago snoring specialist Charles F. Samelson, M.D. Those floppy throat muscles collapse around the tongue, the snorer's airway is completely blocked (halting all sound), and he actually stops breathing for 10, 20, or 30 seconds—or more. These frightening silences happen at regular intervals, often after long sequences of raucous snoring.

After breathing ceases, the snorer's survival instincts usually come to the rescue, and he awakens enough to pull his tongue out of the airway so he can breathe again. As soon as he falls into another deep slumber, however, the process repeats itself.

This malady is called *sleep apnea*. The cause is unknown, although some experts suspect that apnea victims have narrower airways than other snorers. In any case, doctors take the disorder very seriously for several reasons. For one, every year doctors suspect that 2,000 to 3,000 people die in their sleep because of sleep apnea. The deaths are usually caused by suffocation.

And because apnea snorers have to partially wake up at regular intervals to restart their breathing, they spend little of the night in the deep-sleep stages essential for a good rest. That can be particularly dangerous if they're driving or operating machinery on the job. They may also find it harder to learn or grasp complex problems, says Bernard deBerry, M.D., a sleep specialist based in Laguna Hills, California.

But sleepiness isn't the only side effect of sleep apnea. Over the years this nightly stop-and-start breathing can be murder on the snorer's heart because when he stops breathing, his blood becomes depleted of oxygen. So his heart has to labor mightily to circulate blood faster to keep a life-sustaining amount of oxygen going to critical organs like the brain. But the heart wasn't meant to work this hard, and it eventually can become damaged or start to beat irregularly. This makes snorers with sleep apnea more vulnerable to heart attacks and strokes.

And people with sleep apnea are much more likely to suffer from high blood pressure. One study showed that in a group of 1,200 outwardly healthy, working-age men, those with diagnosed sleep apnea were five times as likely to have high blood pressure than those who slept normally. And in another randomly chosen group of 50 men with high blood pressure, 26 percent turned out to have sleep apnea—a much higher percentage than expected in the general population.

So experts say that anyone who has these periods of interrupted breathing during sleep should see a doctor immediately. Sleep apnea is an emergency. The problem, though, is that many apnea snorers deny that their breathing stops every night. Sleep experts say that spouses might have to tape-record the whole frightening apnea cycle to convince "denial snorers" that the problem is real.

What to Do about It

What antisnoring treatment is used depends on what's causing the snore, how much the snorer wants to stop a snoring problem, and how dangerous the snoring is. For a simple snoring problem, doctors often first recommend simple, noninvasive solutions like small changes in lifestyle. If these don't work, the snorer can opt for a surgical procedure or antisnoring device, if it means that much to his quality of life (and his family's). For sleep apnea, doctors frequently suggest surgery or devices first—backed up by the less drastic remedies.

Here's a list of the best antisnoring treatments known, simple and otherwise. (Remember, though, if you suspect that you have sleep apnea—or your bedmate suspects that you do—forgo home remedies and see a doctor without delay.)

Stop drinking alcohol at least three hours before bedtime. Alcohol is also a central nervous system depressant and can have the same effect on throat muscles. In one study at the University of Florida College of Medicine, 20 men who drank one milliliter of 100-proof alcohol per pound of body weight before going to bed (for a 150-pound person, that's about five drinks) had five times as many apneic episodes as they did when they retired sober.

Lose some weight. Snorers are notorious for being overweight, and there's a reason why. When people get fat, they get fat all over—even the throat tissues can swell up. That added bulkiness in the throat can contribute to blocking airways, therefore causing snoring and sleep apnea problems.

Try using a "snore ball." This is a time-honored remedy, designed to keep snorers from sleeping on their backs (which increases the likelihood of snoring). Sew a pocket into the back of the snorer's pajamas, then sew a marble—or even a tennis ball—inside. It will soon encourage the snorer to sleep on his side or stomach.

Avoid tranquilizers, sleeping pills, and antihistamines before bedtime. These central nervous system depressants can cause the muscles in a snorer's throat to become too relaxed and floppy. When this happens, there's more chance of vibration in the airway (and thus more snoring). Plus, the relaxed muscles can cause the tongue to fall backward more easily into the airway.

If stuffy nasal airways are your problem, get them fixed. Sometimes a snoring cure can be as simple as getting a chronically stuffy or blocked-up nose cleared. People with obstructed nasal airways have to really suck in to get air. So they end up creating a vacuum in their throats that pulls together the tissues in the throat so they vibrate more. Medications can clear up blockages caused by nasal allergies or infections. Surgery can correct nasal deformities that may obstruct nasal airways. One common deformity that's easily corrected by surgery is a deviated septum, an irregularity inside the nose in the wall that separates one nostril from the other.

Elevate your head. This strategy helps keep the airway open. The best way to do this is to put a brick or two under the bedposts at the head of the bed. Don't use extra pillows—they'll only kink the airway.

Ask your doctor about a TRD (tongue-retaining device). Available only through sleep centers, a TRD forces the snorer to breathe through his nose by holding the tongue forward and keeping the mouth closed. The tongue-retaining device was developed by Dr. Samelson to treat sleep apnea. In carefully screened apnea patients, he says, a TRD can be effective in eliminating apnea in 82 percent of cases. Though the prescription is written at a sleep disorders center, the device is usually fitted by a dentist.

Ask also about CPAP (continuous positive airway pressure). This is another sleep apnea treatment—a machine that feeds pressurized air to the sleeper through a nose mask, from a bedside tank. As you might imagine, the process can be cumbersome, not to mention inconvenient and uncomfortable. But if a snorer is taught how to use CPAP properly, it can make a real difference. It has about a 90 percent success rate among snorers who use it correctly. If you opt for the CPAP, which some snorers do to avoid surgery, try to get as much help as you can learning to use it.

And ask about UPPP (uvulopalatopharyngoplasty). This is standard surgery for certain victims of both sleep apnea and loud snoring. It's likened to a big tonsillectomy that removes extra throat tissue (like an excessively long palate or uvula, the tissue that dangles in the throat) that could be blocking the airway. Among people who are chosen carefully (which means a thorough evaluation has determined that this extra tissue is causing the snoring or apnea problem), the operation has an 80 percent success rate for snoring. For apnea, the success rate is about 50 percent.

CHAPTER 32

Best Remedies
for Fighting Phlegm

Some expectorants are worth trying—and some are worth forgetting.

How do you talk about . . . er, ah . . . well, phlegm, without sounding disgusting? It isn't easy. But we're going to try because we know you'll thank us later. Like when you're in the throes of your first winter cold, coughing your head off because in your throat and chest is you-know-what.

During a cold or other respiratory infection, mucous membranes (which line your entire respiratory tract) don't release as much liquid as they normally do. So the mucus that is there in the tract changes from its benign, thin, watery consistency to the thick, gross, gummy stuff we call phlegm.

Any aid you use to help you cough up phlegm and get it out of your chest and your life is called by a fancy name: expectorant. Many people think that expectorants work by stimulating your cough reflex so you'll cough more. That extra coughing, they believe, helps bring up the phlegm. "But that's probably not how expectorants operate at all," says pharmacist Branton Lachman, Pharm.D., a University of Southern California School of Pharmacy clinical assistant professor. "Instead, they do their job by attempting to thin out phlegm so it's easier to cough up."

Which expectorants work? That's a hard question to answer, experts say. Expectorants are tough to test under rigorous scientific conditions because everybody's phlegm is different and difficult to measure. Despite these problems, there are some types of expectorants doctors think are worth trying—and some worth forgetting. Here's a rundown.

Extra fluids: from water to chicken soup. Almost every expert we consulted said that extra fluids were the most effective expectorants to reach for, especially as a first line of defense. "Extra fluids go into all compartments of the body, including your respiratory tract, where they help to liquefy hardened mucus so it's easier to cough up," says Dr. Lachman. How much extra fluid is enough? Dr. Lachman recommends six to eight eight-ounce glasses a day, which includes your usual amount. (Patients on fluid restriction should check with their physicians first.)

Does chicken soup, that oldest of folk remedies for a cold, have any magical qualities as an expectorant? Probably not, say our experts, although it's a delicious, nutritious way to take in extra fluids. One famous study, conducted at Mount Sinai Medical Center in Miami Beach, Florida, found that chicken soup made volunteers' noses run faster than did other hot or cold liquids. But the researchers didn't attempt to measure the soup's effect on phlegm deeper in the respiratory tract, the kind that needs to be coughed up.

And what about that oft-quoted piece of wisdom that says to avoid drinking milk during a cold because it increases the amount of phlegm in your system? Not true, says Dr. Lachman. "Milk does not produce phlegm, infection does," he says. Why do so many people think milk is a phlegm producer? "It may be because milk is a coating liquid. It gives you the feeling of more phlegm in your throat, but the milk isn't really increasing the amount."

Vaporizers and humidifiers. Some doctors also recommend humidifying the air you breathe to help thin mucus. Other doctors say you have to drink extra fluids for humidifying devices to have an effect on deep-down congestion—just breathing in moisture through the air isn't enough. Since moistened air can keep dry nasal passages comfortable, however, there's certainly no harm in keeping a humidifier going during a cold.

Camphor-menthol chest rubs. The Food and Drug Administration (FDA) says it doesn't have enough information to rate camphor-menthol chest rubs, such as Vicks VapoRub, as effective expectorants. But it did recently decide that camphor and menthol can individually be effective to calm a cough. So if you're coughing a lot, and all that hacking is unproductive (that is, you're not getting up phlegm with your coughing), you might use one of these rubs, especially at night so you can sleep better. One caution, however: Chest rubs should never be taken internally in any amount.

Other home remedies. Lozenges containing licorice, horehound, or aromatic oils such as peppermint or spearmint are often linked with increased breakdown of phlegm, says Varro E. Tyler, Ph.D., a professor of pharmacognosy (the study of drugs derived from animals and plants) at Purdue University. As they dissolve in your throat, they help liquefy mucus, he says.

And hot, spicy foods—the kind that make your eyes water or your nose run—may also be modestly effective. "They help mucous membranes all over, not just in your

nose, to secrete more liquid, which can help thin mucus,"
Dr. Tyler says. So you might want to add foods containing
hot peppers, curry, and other hot and spicy flavorings to
your menu when you have a cold. If you're not used to
such foods, be careful to use them sparingly at first.
"There's a great deal of difference in the sensitivities of
people's palates when it comes to things like hot peppers—
so be cautious," says Dr. Tyler.

Over-the-counter drugs. The most common expectorant
ingredient in most over-the-counter cough remedies is guaifenesin (found in some formulations of Robitussin, Be-
nylin, Sudafed, Triaminic, and other products advertised
as containing expectorants). Guaifenesin stimulates your
stomach to release body fluids that are supposed to travel
to your chest and go to work to thin out phlegm. But does
it really do the job?

Many experts think that studies have been inconclusive
about whether guaifenesin actually does have an effect on
phlegm. But apparently the FDA begs to differ. Sources at
the FDA say that it has analyzed new evidence about
guaifenesin's effectiveness and that the agency is "likely"
to move the drug into its "safe and effective" category as
an over-the-counter expectorant sometime later this year.
Up until now, the FDA has said it didn't have enough
evidence to make a decision on guaifenesin's effectiveness.

If guaifenesin's status does change, it will be the one
and only expectorant the FDA categorizes this way. The
agency has judged all other over-the-counter expectorants
as either not effective or not tested enough to provide
evidence to rule one way or the other.

What about cough medicines that combine expectorants
with other cold remedies? Many doctors and pharmacists
would probably be reluctant to recommend such combination drugs if all you need is an expectorant. But a lot of
physicians would also agree that in some situations a
cough suppressant-expectorant combination is justified.
"Some people may have an incredibly sensitive cough
reflex, which the suppressant could help tone down so
they're not coughing all the time," says Dr. Lachman.
"Then, if the expectorant is doing its job, you'll only cough
when there's something actually ready to be coughed up."

Exercise. If you're careful to wait until the acute stage of your cold is over (after you're through battling the infection and your temperature is normal again), exercise just might help you loosen up phlegm left in your respiratory tract. So say several experts, including Bryant Stamford, Ph.D., director of the Health Promotion and Wellness Center, University of Louisville School of Medicine. "It may be that the jarring effect of exercise helps to break up mucus," he says.

Whatever expectorant you use, it's a good idea to see a doctor if you keep coughing up a lot of phlegm for several days. You could have a more serious respiratory infection, such as pneumonia. Also, any cough that's unrelated to a cold, or a cough that seems to be getting better, then gets worse again, should be checked out by a professional.

CHAPTER 33

Help for Heel Pain

by Stephen Lally

Sometimes simple rest is all you need.

My heel problems all started when I went out dancing in my supertraction boat moccasins. I went at the last minute, and I didn't think about changing my shoes. So when I got on the dance floor, I tried to overcompensate. It didn't work. I twisted my ankle.

For the rest of the weekend, I did smart things. I treated my injury by following the RICE method: rested the foot, iced the sore spot, compressed the area with a makeshift Ace bandage, and elevated the foot on a chair as I watched TV. My ankle felt better, but a little sore. For the next couple of weeks, I kept my weight toward the outside edge of my foot to baby the injury. And that minor change in my stride is what finally sent me to the podiatrist—with a royal pain (ouch!) in my heel.

My situation was unusual. My heel injury was not. The

podiatrist told me I had *plantar fasciitis* (PLAN-tar fassy-EYE-tiss), probably the single most common cause of heel pain.

The *plantar fascia* (FAS-see-uh) is a ligament-like piece of connective tissue on the bottom of the foot. It runs the length of the arch, from the five metatarsal bones in front to the heel bone in back.

The fascia is not very stretchable—and that's where your heel problems can begin. Walking normally, your arch stretches and flattens a little with every step. Your foot rolls in slightly as well. Podiatrists call that *pronation*. Any movement that overpronates puts stress on the arch and on the plantar fascia. If this happens repeatedly, the fascia begins to tear or pull away from the heel bone, and the whole area becomes inflamed. Plantar fasciitis is afoot. In time, it hurts—a lot!

But the sneakiest aspect of plantar fasciitis is that, at first, it doesn't feel like anything serious. In fact, for a while you might not feel anything at all. (I was an exception. I had a mild pulling sensation down the length of my arch, like a stretching rubber band.) When the pain does begin, it concentrates in a small spot on the inner front of the heel, just behind the highest part of the arch. "People describe it as a 'stone bruise' that won't go away," says Joe Ellis, D.P.M., a podiatrist and consultant to the University of California, San Diego. "It's usually annoying, but they'll put up with it for weeks. That's how it gets worse."

Another telltale sign: pain that's worse in the morning, when you first stand on the affected foot. That happens because the fascia is being newly stressed after an overnight rest. As you walk around, the fascia gradually "warms up" and lengthens slightly. That reduces the tension: Less pull means less pain. But after several weeks, the pain doesn't go away as quickly. And the worse it gets, the longer it will take to cure the problem.

Deterring Pain

Plantar fasciitis is an overuse injury, which means it can happen to anyone who repeatedly overstresses a foot. "You can be a gold-medal Olympian in perfect shape, training 15 miles a day. One day you push hard to 16. Or you can be a 350-pound couch potato who gets off his butt and walks 1 mile. In each case, if that extra mile is more than your feet can take, you'll get an overuse injury," says Jeff Bronson, M.D., an orthopedic surgeon in San Diego. People who run or do high-impact aerobics are more likely to overstress their plantar fascia. But anybody who begins an exercise program (even walking) and does too much too soon is at risk.

But no one is doomed to get plantar fasciitis. Several careful studies of injured runners revealed little evidence that anatomical differences were at the root of overuse problems. Out of several studies, only one physical marker has been consistently associated with a greater risk of plantar fasciitis: being able to flex your foot downward (bending at the ankle and pointing your toes down) more than 60 degrees. "You can't measure that accurately at home—and you may not need to worry about it anyway," says Stephen P. Messier, Ph.D., director of the J. B. Snow Biomechanics Laboratory at Wake Forest University in Winston-Salem, North Carolina, "since many people with that degree of flexibility don't get heel pain."

The bottom line: Plantar fasciitis is avoidable, if you don't do more than your feet can handle. An overuse injury is a self-inflicted wound. The best way to avoid it: Know your limits. Work up slowly to new milestones. Know when to quit for the day. And wear the right shoes with good cushioning, shock-absorbing capability and stability.

Giving Your Injured Foot a Hand

Okay, let's say you've been dancing in boat shoes, and you're hurting now. If your pain fits the two telltale signs— (1) it's concentrated in the front of the heel pad and (2) it's worse in the morning or after a long rest period—then you've probably got plantar fasciitis. You may want to check with a podiatrist to make sure it's not something else. Then you can try some of the simple self-help methods listed below. Reliable podiatrists will recommend that you try these low-tech methods before they suggest surgery or custom-made orthotic shoe inserts.

Give the foot a rest. Fasciitis is, after all, an overuse injury. If you've been running or walking farther than usual, cut back to half your distance. Better yet, rest for a week or two, then come back slowly. If you've just started to get a tender spot, you may get over it in a few weeks. But if you've had pain for a while, don't expect miracles. It took me about six months to get over my fasciitis completely.

Try other forms of exercise. Simply varying your workout with a less foot-dependent sport might be all you need in the early stages of fasciitis. Swimming is an excellent substitute.

Take a nonsteroidal anti-inflammatory. As the name says, these drugs reduce inflammation and so decrease pain. Follow instructions for seven to ten days, and take medication after eating to reduce stomach upset.

Massage the painful area with ice. This is another good way to reduce inflammation. Once or twice a day for no more than 20 minutes at a time should suffice.

Stretch your Achilles tendon. Crazy as it sounds, this works! That's because a tight Achilles tendon, which runs from the bottom of the heel to the calf muscle, pulls the heel bone up and back, stressing the fascia. A more relaxed tendon and calf muscle puts less strain on the injury. Here's one good stretching technique: Stand facing a wall, with one leg in front of the other. Keeping the back foot flat on the ground, bend the front leg slowly at the knee. Balance yourself against the wall as you lean forward. Keep the back leg straight. You'll feel a pulling in the calf muscle and Achilles tendon. Hold 20 to 30 seconds. Switch legs and repeat.

Wear shoes with good arch and heel support. Running shoes and the newer "pro" walking shoes are excellent choices. Don't skimp! "There's a big difference between the support you get from the $50 shoe and the $11 shoe that's supposed to look like the $50 shoe," says Dr. Bronson. Arch support helps prevent overpronation. Solid heel support prevents the heel from pressing down too hard and therefore putting too much pressure on the fascia. I was able to wear my running shoes most of the time— even at work. If you can't, try the next alternative.

Buy nonprescription arch supports. These are relatively

inexpensive and can be switched from one pair of shoes to another. Sometimes they come with an extra metatarsal pad under the ball of the foot. Peel that off—it won't help fasciitis. My supports were great when I had to wear dress shoes. I even wore the supports in my running shoes! That felt a little strange at first, but it helped a lot. I still use them once in a while, because they feel so good.

Have your foot taped by someone who knows what they're doing. Two styles of taping, the *heel lock* and *low-dye taping,* can reduce overpronation. "But it's really difficult to tape your own foot effectively for this condition," says Dr. Ellis. "An athletic trainer from a local college can do a good job. Amateurs have a tough time."

Try all of the above. Try various combinations of these simple therapies, and give them time. You should start to feel some improvement in a week or so, if you've caught the problem early. If you've had pain for a while, be patient.

There are several things you shouldn't try:

- Don't apply heat. It won't help fasciitis.
- Don't use a foot soak. Again, it won't do much. You can soak your foot in cool water (about 50°F) for 20 minutes as an alternative to ice massage. But the ice is better, since it can be held directly on the sore spot.
- Don't expect extra padding or heel cups to solve the problem. The injury is caused by overstretching, not impact. A heel cup or pad might feel better, but that's because it relieves pressure on the inflamed area. Extra cushioning won't stop the stretching.

What the Doctor Can Do

When these simple measures fail—if you don't notice any improvement after a month or two, or if your improvement has leveled off—it's time to visit a podiatrist, orthopedic surgeon, or sports medicine specialist. A professional can provide four things that you can't.

Cortisone injections. It's not pleasant, but an injection of this anti-inflammatory drug directly into the sore spot can provide powerful relief for a few days. Be careful, though. There are two main types of cortisone: water soluble and fat soluble (also called insoluble). Since long-term exposure to cortisone can actually damage the fascia, make sure the specialist is using the water-soluble variety, or a mixture of the two. To be safe, don't have cortisone injections done more than three times in the same foot.

Advanced physical therapy. Under the guidance of a physical therapist, you can learn a regimen of ice massage, friction massage, and stretching exercises. Or you can be given ultrasound treatments, in which sound waves are used to massage the fascia, break up scar tissue, and promote healing.

Custom orthotic shoe inserts. Orthotics are high-tech supports for the entire foot. To achieve a custom fit, the doctor makes a cast impression of your feet. The orthotics are then molded out of any one of a variety of materials. Semirigid materials such as polypropylene are probably the best, since they provide support without being hard on your feet.

Orthotics are a mixed bag. On the plus side, a good pair can provide permanent relief. On the minus side, they are expensive: anywhere from $300 to $1,000 per pair. (It pays to shop around, since a higher price doesn't always mean better quality.)

But when they work, they can be worth every penny. Some people wear them for a few months, take them out, and never have pain again. Others have to wear orthotics for life. While most orthotics are very good, there are no guarantees. Sometimes it takes weeks for the pain to go away. And an unfortunate few don't get relief from orthotics. They are the only people who should consider surgery.

Fascia release operation. In most cases, this is relatively simple outpatient surgery done under local anesthesia. The surgeon cuts into the side of the heel and snips partway (up to one inch) through the fascia to release the area being pulled. Contrary to popular belief, this surgery won't leave you with flat feet. Once the site of the operation heals, the pain is usually gone. And major complications are rare. As Dr. Ellis reports, "I performed this operation on a former Olympic miler. Five weeks later, he went running. The first time out, he thought he felt a twinge. Since then, he's had no problems."

It sounds wonderful, but it truly should be a last resort. As with any surgery, there is a risk of infection and minor nerve damage. The heel can swell excessively and heal slowly—keeping you off your feet even longer. And the resulting scar tissue may thicken over time and cause a recurrence of pain. These complications occur in about 15 percent of cases.

One operation that won't help plantar fasciitis is heel spur removal. A few years ago, these bony growths were popularly thought to be the cause of heel pain, and many were removed unnecessarily. Actually, the spurs aren't a cause, but an effect. The bone reacts to the pulling of the fascia by growing outward. "A good number of people who have heel spurs feel no pain, and many cases of plantar fasciitis are not accompanied by spur formation," says Suzanne M. Tanner, M.D., a sports medicine physician in Denver and an alumna of the prestigious Hughston Sports Clinic.

How My Heel Healed

My podiatrist gave me a cortisone shot, a variety of felt-material arch supports, a heel cup, and the advice to stay off my foot as much as possible. The shot was momentarily unpleasant, but it helped. The arch supports felt like they did me the most good. When they wore out, I bought nonprescription supports in a drugstore. I never tried the heel cup. I truly did try to follow the advice and succeeded about half the time. But when you have an overuse injury in a part of the body you can't avoid using, healing time will be unbearably slow. Your best course is to use common sense, try the simple remedies if possible, and have plenty of patience.

It took me six months to do it, but now I'm completely pain free. Anybody wanna go dancing?

CHAPTER 34

Antihistamine Advice
That Won't
Start You Snoring

You may have to try a dozen brands, but almost everyone can find better, nondrowsy relief.

Three-quarters of allergic individuals admit that they take their allergy medications less than half the time they experience symptoms, reports a national survey of over 1,000 adults conducted by the Opinion Research Corporation of Princeton, New Jersey. The reason? Reduced alertness.

Unfortunately, experts feel that antihistamines have to be taken on a regular basis (or at least at the first tingle of emerging symptoms) to be effective. So all of those skipped pills add up to poor control of symptoms, they say.

But all antihistamines are not alike, and there aren't just a few to choose among, either.

Many physicians feel that for almost everyone, somewhere there lurks an antihistamine that can drop symptoms down into low gear without downshifting the brain as well.

How They Do What They Do

"The exact reason that antihistamines work is unknown," explains Anthony J. Ricketti, M.D., former clinical associate professor of medicine at Rutgers Medical School. "But many of them bear a physical resemblance to histamine itself."

Histamine is one of the chemicals released by your body during an allergic reaction. Release of histamine "turns

239

on" your allergy symptoms, such as hives, runny nose, itchy eyes, and so on.

"This resemblance," says Dr. Ricketti, "has led to the speculation that antihistamines may 'compete' with histamine."And that, explains Dr. Ricketti, is why antihistamines can't do anything about the symptoms that any released histamine has already caused. "They can only prevent more histamine from binding and causing new, or worsening, symptoms.

"Antihistamines," he adds, "are most useful in controlling symptoms like itching and rhinorrhea [a runny nose]. They are less effective in relieving nasal obstruction and allergic eye problems."

Sheldon L. Spector, M.D., a clinical professor of medicine at the University of California, Los Angeles, agrees. He feels that antihistamines do some of their best work relieving the allergic itch.

"Antihistamines alleviate the itching and hives that the histamine released during an allergic reaction can produce," he explains. "They are the treatment of choice for bad cases of hives and are the main therapy for people with chronic hives."

Seldane Socks Sleepiness

There is an antihistamine available with a different composition that doesn't make people drowsy. Its generic name is terfenadine, and it is sold under the brand name Seldane in the United States. It's been shown to be as effective as "regular" antihistamines in many studies and is available with a doctor's prescription.

A variety of other nonsedating antihistamines are just itching to hit the U.S. market. Some are still in the early stages of development; others have been used (some as over-the-counter drugs) in other countries for years.

But many physicians say that Seldane and its emerging cousins are not your only choice for nonsedating allergy relief. It's their experience that most people can use a pick-and-choose method and eventually find an antihistamine that shuts down only the symptoms—and not the sufferer.

"People who turn to Seldane may have only tried one

regular antihistamine first, had a bad experience, and thought that the problem—drowsiness, stomach upset— was true of all antihistamines," says Dr. Spector.

"But of course, it's not—people can react very differently to the different varieties available. Many of my patients have been able to find a regular antihistamine they can use without feeling sleepy.

"Seldane works great, but it doesn't work for everyone, and you can frequently get the same level of relief and lack of sedation by shopping around with traditional antihistamines," he says.

Pick a Pack

"I let the person with the symptoms decide which antihistamine works best for them," explains Mark E. Demichiei, M.D., an assistant clinical professor of family medicine at the Medical College of Ohio.

"I give each of my patients about seven different samples that include at least one variety from each of the five major classes. They try each one for two days and keep track of how each works on their symptoms and whether it causes any side effects, such as drowsiness or stomach upset.

"I've found there's no way to predict people's reactions to antihistamines. Both the level of relief and the side effects they cause are so individualized that there's no single one I can recommend to people. But invariably," he asserts, "they'll find one that makes them feel better without making them tired or nauseated."

And finding that drug, he says, is essential for people who can't otherwise control their allergy symptoms. "There's no question about taking antihistamines continuously," says Dr. Demichiei. "It's definitely a drug that works better when taken for prevention than after symptoms have already developed.

"And to get people to do that, you've got to help them find a drug that they can live with. My patients generally leave my office with at least a two-week supply of samples, but if they find one that they're satisfied with, they don't have to go through the remainder."

It's a system that many allergists endorse. Kurt von

Maur, M.D., associate clinical professor of medicine at the College of Human Medicine of Michigan State University, reports that only 7 out of 758 of his patients (that's less than 1 percent) were unable to find an antihistamine that took care of their symptoms without intolerable side effects.

He gave each of his patients five different "starter packs" and had them record their symptoms and side effects while taking each one for two weeks. Once they picked a final choice, he notes, they generally stayed with it. At the end of a year, 78 percent were still using that antihistamine.

Although several studies and reference works have attempted to rate the many different classes, subclasses, and varieties of antihistamines according to their effectiveness and incidence of side effects, the results are often downright contradictory.

Experts emphasize that individual reactions to these drugs vary greatly. You might be put to sleep by one study's "least sedating" variety or energized by an antihistamine that puts most other people to sleep when they just think about taking it.

Talk to your doctor to be sure that there isn't any reason for you to avoid antihistamines. Get a bunch of samples and/or pick up a variety of over-the-counter versions. Keep a record of each one's effectiveness and side effects, using a homemade chart. Then pick the one that does the most for your symptoms while taking away the least of your alertness.

Combinations: Can They "Cancel Out" Side Effects?

Many antihistamines are also available in combination with another active ingredient, a decongestant. While antihistamines have a tendency to make people sleepy, decongestants do the opposite.

Combining the two, feel many physicians, often cancels out the unwanted side effects (sleepiness on one hand, jittery alertness on the other) of each.

Dr. Demichiei says that most of his patients tend to choose combinations. But he asks, "Are they using combination products because they cancel out the side effects— or because of the extra relief that the decongestant provides? Most people *are* going to feel like they're getting more relief with a combination product."

Dr. von Maur feels that the passage of time, like decongestants, may also reduce antihistamine-induced drowsiness.

"Drowsiness with antihistamines tends to diminish after you've been taking the medication for a while," he explains. "But luckily, the effectiveness *doesn't* diminish along with the drowsiness."

Of Course, Drug-Free Is Best—But . . .

Allergy experts make it perfectly clear that antihistamines should *not* be the only way a person handles an allergy. They advocate environmental controls and limiting exposure to your allergy trigger as a first line of defense.

But such controls are easier for some allergy aggravators—pets and house dust, for instance—than for things that are often impossible to avoid, such as molds and pollen. (You can't stay inside *all* spring and fall!)

And don't neglect the positive side of side effects either. Drowsiness, points out Dr. Spector, isn't such a bad thing when it's time to go to bed. Some of his patients like to use a very effective but somewhat sleep-inducing antihistamine at night and then switch to a different variety or a combination product in the morning.

(However, Dr. Spector does *not* advocate the use of antihistamines as sleep inducers alone. Allergies, he points out, are the only reason to take them.)

Flash Reports

GETTING THE BEST
BREAST CANCER THERAPY

A recent alert from the National Cancer Institute reported the preliminary results of three unpublished studies on breast cancer treatment. The studies looked at women with breast cancer that had not spread to their lymph nodes. It found that in these women, both surgery *and* chemotherapy or hormone treatment generally provided longer cancer-free survival time than the usual surgery-only treatment. (The supplemental treatment was started no more than six to eight weeks after surgery.)

Does this mean that every woman who's had breast cancer surgery should also have chemotherapy or hormone treatment? Experts say no. It *does* mean these women need to make sure they get appropriate additional treatment if they need it. That's not something that automatically happens, says former National Cancer Institute director Vincent DeVita, M.D.

So how do you make sure you're one of the women who gets maximum appropriate care? At the very least, you can ask your doctor to explain the rationale for treatment and consider getting a second opinion. But the most important step is to ask a tumor specialist (oncologist), your surgeon, or a radiotherapist to review your medical records. This advice applies even if you had breast cancer surgery years ago.

You can also ask your doctor to test the tumor for estrogen receptors, a procedure that can help determine if you need hormone therapy. And before surgery, you may want to ask about checking your tumor with *DNA flow cytometry.* This sophisticated new test appears promising in determining a tumor's ability to spread, and it may help your doctor make an accurate decision regarding chemotherapy. It's available in only a few commercial laboratories.

THE PILL: EXERCISE CAUTION

Recently a California gynecologist noted that his patients with functional ovarian cysts had a common connection. All were taking multiphasic birth control pills. These pills, in which the amount of estrogen varies during the monthly cycle, are considered among the safest, especially for older women. In fact, until now, all oral contraceptives have been thought to *reduce* the risk of functional ovarian cysts because they suppress ovulation.

Since his findings were published in the *American Journal of Obstetrics and Gynecology,* the doctor, James Caillouette, M.D., says he has gotten calls nationwide from other doctors noticing the same connection.

Just how risky are these pills? Unfortunately, there's no firm answer. Dr. Caillouette thinks women who get a functional cyst may be able to avoid surgery if they discontinue use of the triphasic pill (three different dosages throughout the month) and switch to a monophasic type (one dosage only).

BLOOD PRESSURE DRUG PRESERVES POTENCY

Many blood pressure drugs can send a man's sex life into a tailspin. They may reduce sexual desire or make it difficult for him to maintain an erection or to ejaculate.

A new study, though, found one hypertension drug that *doesn't* cause these problems. It's captopril, an angiotensin converting enzyme (ACE) inhibitor.

The study, from researchers at the University of Connecticut Health Center, involved 626 hypertensive men who took one of three blood pressure drugs, with or without diuretics: captopril; methyldopa, a central nervous system depressant; or propranolol, a beta-blocker. Anonymous questionnaires used to report sexual symptoms before and during treatment showed that only men treated with captopril retained their usual sexual functioning. Those taking a diuretic along with methyldopa or propranolol had the most sexual problems.

Often, simply switching to captopril stops sexual problems caused by other hypertension drugs, these researchers report. And they say many people with what's known as primary hypertension do well on the drug.

ULTRA PROSTATE CARE
WITH ULTRASOUND

Ultrasound, the same painless technique that can outline a fetus in the womb, is now being used to examine and treat the prostate gland. Ultrasound imaging of the prostate is obtained by inserting a sound-emitting probe into the rectum. The image can be recorded on laser disk, enabling doctors to track changes over the years. (Cancer diagnosis still requires a nearly painless tissue biopsy.)

Ultrasound imaging is also being used in the treatment of prostate cancer to help direct the placement of cancer-killing radioactive "seeds." This new treatment reduces the risk of nerve damage and impaired sexual function associated with prostate surgery.

CHAPTER 35

Uterine Fibroids:
Clear Up Your Confusion

Unfortunately, no one knows yet how to prevent these benign tumors. But here's the inside story on what treatments doctors recommend.

Over age 30, more than 20 percent of women have fibroid tumors, also known as leiomyomas or fibromyomas, benign growths of muscle and connective tissue in the uterus. Many women are unaware of their fibroids until the growths are discovered during pelvic exam. Fibroids may grow large enough to change the shape of the uterus and compromise fertility. For unknown reasons, black women suffer three times more fibroids than white women.

A Case of Tissue Overgrowth

The uterus is composed of densely packed muscle fibers. Estrogen and growth hormone encourage overgrowth of these fibers, which is why fibroids grow rapidly during pregnancy and usually regress after menopause. Estrogen birth control pills can also encourage fibroid growth, but the newer low-dose pills do not. Postmenopausal estrogen may also induce fibroid growth, so dosage should be kept to a minimum.

Fibroids can form on the inside or outside of the uterus. Outside tumors can be felt more easily by a clinician. A woman can sometimes feel them herself by lying flat, relaxing her abdomen, and pressing down in the area just above the pubic hair line. Fibroids feel firm and irregular in shape. These external fibroids can grow so large they fill much of the abdomen and crowd the bladder and rectum. If they outgrow their blood supply, fibroids can cause severe pelvic pain.

Fibroids inside the uterus can bulge into the uterine cavity, distorting the space and causing heavy and erratic menstrual periods. Anemia and pain can result.

A woman with fibroids may have difficulty becoming pregnant, especially if the growths are large. Fibroid removal, or myomectomy, restores fertility, but the growths may return. Pregnant women with fibroids have an increased risk of miscarriage during the first and second trimester. They may also experience severe pain due to rapid fibroid growth and may require hospitalization for proper diagnosis.

Treatment for Fibroids

If you or your clinician suspect you have uterine fibroids, their size can be assessed by ultrasound examination, an imaging technique that does not carry the radiation hazard of x-rays. If your fibroids appear to be growing rapidly, request an ultrasound exam every 6 to 12 months.

If fibroids cause heavy periods, drink lots of fluids, take iron tablets daily, and have a blood test at least twice a year to ensure you're not becoming anemic. Since heavy bleeding can indicate a number of serious gynecological problems, have your condition checked thoroughly by your clinician.

Many doctors recommend hysterectomy, surgical removal of the uterus. A myomectomy, which removes the fibroids but retains the uterus, is a good alternative. With a myomectomy, a woman retains her fertility and sexual responsiveness, which some women lose after hysterectomy. Compared with hysterectomy, myomectomy also causes less risk of premenopausal heart attack. The disadvantage of this surgery is that the fibroids may grow back.

For postmenopausal women whose fibroids are growing rapidly, hysterectomy is usually recommended. In rare cases, fibroids may be cancerous, usually in women over age 50.

Although not yet widely available, there are new treatments for fibroids that cause heavy bleeding. One is a surgical technique called ablation of the endometrium, in which the uterine lining that bleeds every month is permanently removed by laser or surgical excision. The uterus is retained and the procedure does not involve any abdominal incisions, since it is performed through the vagina.

Other new treatments under investigation lower estrogen levels. One being tested by Latin American and European researchers involves an experimental drug, gestinone, that lowers estrogen and progesterone blood levels, terminates menstrual periods, and shrinks fibroids. Another treatment involves a newly synthesized brain hormone, gonadotropic releasing hormone (GnRH), which also reduces hormone levels and stops the periods.

Unfortunately, we don't know enough about the causes of uterine fibroids to prevent them. To give yourself the best protection, use only low-dose birth control pills or, preferably, other means of contraception. If you are postmenopausal and have fibroids, avoid estrogen treatments. Although researchers are unsure whether diet can decrease or eliminate fibroids, you might try eating a vegetarian diet high in fibrous plant material, which is known to decrease blood estrogen levels.

CHAPTER 36

What Every Woman Should Know about Hysterectomy

New technology is bringing us new options.

Debra, 46, a real-estate developer, had a fibroid inside her uterus for four years. It didn't cause any problems until two years ago, when her periods became heavier, "until I was bleeding half the month. Then, I flew overseas, and because of the change in air pressure, I nearly bled to death."

Her gynecologist's advice: Have a hysterectomy.

Instead, she found a physician skilled at a procedure that removes the fibroid but not the uterus. "I went into the hospital in the morning. When I came out of anesthesia, I had about a minute of pain. I was out of the recovery room at 1:00 P.M. and walked out of the hospital at 3:00 P.M. I had no painkillers afterward. Two days later, I was back at work, with no more bleeding."

Debra said no to hysterectomy; she explored her options before surgery and found what was, for her, a better solution.

A smart move? Women's health advocates say yes, absolutely. Getting a second opinion—and checking out alternative treatments—is always important when you face major elective surgery. And, in the case of hysterectomy (removal of the uterus), it may be especially critical.

One in every three women will face hysterectomy. In the United States alone, over 654,000 women had the surgery last year. About 45 percent of them had their ovaries removed, too, in a procedure called oophorectomy.

Those numbers have remained fairly constant over the last ten years, despite growing concern among some physicians and consumer groups that many hysterectomies are unnecessary.

Nora W. Coffey, president of the HERS (Hysterectomy Educational Resources and Services) Foundation —a Pennsylvania-based nonprofit organization that offers support and counseling for women who have had or are contemplating hysterectomy—believes that in many cases the surgery is avoidable. "Of the women we sent for second opinions, 98 percent did not have to have hysterectomies after treatment by a specialist for their specific symptoms," she contends.

George W. Morley, M.D., chairman of the American College of Obstetricians and Gynecologists task force on hysterectomy, has a more moderate view. "Sure, there are unindicated hysterectomies—we know that—but I don't think the percentage is particularly high," he says.

In truth, there's no way to determine exactly how many

women who have had hysterectomies or are headed for one really need it. One thing's for sure, however: The numbers aren't very reassuring. Researchers can't explain, for example, why Southerners undergo nearly twice as many hysterectomies as Yankees. Even within states, there are inexplicable variations. And hysterectomy rates in the United States are two to three times higher than in France and Britain. People have to wonder why.

Another reason to be cautious: Hysterectomy carries with it all the usual risks of major surgery—and possibly more. Physicians say most women don't experience problems. But studies do show that hysterectomy is associated with depression more frequently than other major surgery. Since she founded HERS in 1982, Coffey claims she's counseled thousands of women suffering from depression, as well as a wide range of other long-term posthysterectomy (and/or postoophorectomy) problems, including loss of sexual desire, joint pain, insomnia, weight gain, urinary problems, and fatigue. Research suggests that hysterectomy—even without oophorectomy—may increase risk of heart disease, early ovarian failure, bone loss, and sexual dysfunction. Unfortunately, the research in these areas remains inconsistent and inconclusive. But it does raise some serious concerns.

When to Say Yes

This is not to say you should avoid a hysterectomy at all costs. Everyone agrees that, in the case of invasive cancer, a hysterectomy may be a woman's best chance for survival. (Cancerous conditions account for about 10 percent of hysterectomies.) Similarly, hysterectomy during childbirth or other surgical procedures, when bleeding can't be stopped any other way, can be a lifesaving necessity.

Eighty percent of hysterectomies are done for problems like fibroids, uterine prolapse, and endometriosis, which are not life threatening. In these cases, hysterectomy should be considered as a last resort when other forms of treatment have failed.

As Debra discovered, today there are more alternatives to hysterectomy than ever before. Keep in mind, however, some are controversial; they may or may not be appropriate in your situation, and they all carry risks of their own. But they're worth considering. And for some they may offer a sound reason to say no to hysterectomy.

For Fibroids

Uterine fibroids are hard knots of muscle fiber that grow inward or outward from the muscular wall of the uterus. About a third of women over age 35 have them. They're also the number one indication for hysterectomy, accounting for 41 percent of those done on women aged 35 to 54.

Watchful waiting is most often the best course of action. If you have fibroids but no symptoms, you probably don't need a hysterectomy, says Dr. Morley. "Fibroids alone are not an indication for hysterectomy. But the symptoms or signs related to fibroids may be an indication."

Although most uterine fibroids don't cause problems, they can trigger bleeding or grow large enough to affect the bladder, kidneys, or other organs. A rapidly growing fibroid should be carefully monitored because of the very rare chance that it could be cancerous. Keep in mind, however, that fewer than $^1/_{10}$ of 1 percent of fibroids are cancerous; these are usually found in menopausal women over age 50.

Conventional medical wisdom once held that a fibroid uterus larger than the size of a 14-to-16-week pregnancy should be removed, but that's now disputed. Dr. Morley says he would draw the line at a 17-to-20-week size. "A fibroid has to be pretty big to put pressure on the other organs." Francis Hutchins, Jr., M.D., clinical associate professor at Hahnemann Hospital in Philadelphia, believes that the decision to remove a fibroid uterus is very individual. "I have let a six-month-sized uterus alone, since the symptoms were not debilitating," he says.

Watchful waiting is a particularly good idea if a woman is approaching menopause. Fibroids are fueled by estrogen, which dwindles after menopause, notes gynecologist Ruth Schwartz, M.D., professor at the University of Rochester School of Medicine in New York.

A disappearing ovary (obscured by an enlarged uterus)

is not reason enough to remove the uterus. Women are sometimes frightened into unnecessary hysterectomy when they are told that their fibroids make it difficult for the doctor to feel the ovaries for cancer, says Dr. Morley.

Ovarian cancer is a rare but often deadly disease, affecting less than 2 percent of all women.

"Today we can use ultrasound and CAT scanning to assess the ovaries," says Dr. Morley. "For the uterus to be so big that the ovaries cannot be assessed, it probably has to be the size of a four-to-five-month pregnancy. Otherwise, if you can't feel the ovaries or see them on ultrasound, they probably aren't very big—and that's probably a good sign."

Sadja Greenwood, M.D., a general practitioner long associated with women's health programs and assistant clinical professor at the University of California, San Francisco, Medical Center, agrees. "If you know someone has an unusual ovary, you wouldn't wait to act. But if someone tells a patient, 'We better take this fibroid out in case your ovaries become cancerous,' that's unnecessary surgery."

Simpler surgical procedures may be available. If fibroids must be removed, the surgery needn't be a hysterectomy. "A lot of pelvic surgery that formerly required opening the abdomen now can be done through a hysteroscope or, rarely, a laparoscope to remove small tumors causing bleeding," notes Dr. Hutchins. But not all surgeons are familiar with these relatively quick, lower-risk techniques.

A hysteroscope is a telescope-like instrument that's inserted through the vagina into the uterus and is used to cut off small fibroids or polyps. (This is the surgery that helped Debra.) The laparoscope, which is inserted through a small incision in the abdomen, can be used to detect and then remove fibroids on the outside of the uterus. These fibroids rarely cause problems, however.

Improved techniques enable qualified doctors to remove large fibroids while leaving the uterus intact. Another alternative to hysterectomy is a myomectomy, which involves removing fibroids by opening the abdomen and uterus. In France, myomectomy is routine for fibroids, and the uterus is removed only as a last resort.

U.S. physicians have traditionally avoided myomectomy. It's major surgery, with a complication rate slightly higher than for hysterectomy. Risks include bleeding to the point of transfusion in a fifth of women. In about 10 to 30 percent of cases, fibroids regrow after myomectomy.

But techniques are improving, says Dr. Hutchins, and a skilled surgeon should have complication rates no higher than for hysterectomy. Capable physicians can often be found at reputable fertility clinics, he adds.

If you're very near to menopause, hormonal treatments may help tide you over until nature takes its course. There are several hormonal therapies that can shut off estrogen temporarily, to shrink fibroids in preparation for surgery or until menopause, notes gynecologist Andrew J. Friedman, M.D., assistant professor at the Harvard Medical School. One treatment is gonadotropic releasing hormone (GnRH) agonist, which stops the ovaries from producing estrogen, shrinking fibroids dramatically. (GnRH is an approved treatment for certain prostate problems; Food and Drug Administration approval for its use in treating gynecological problems is expected in the near future.)

GnRH can cause menopausal symptoms, such as hot flashes and vaginal dryness. In a minority of women, there are more severe side effects, such as muscle and joint stiffness, headaches, hair loss, swelling, and fatigue. Bone density drops on GnRH. And although this is reversible, GnRH should not be used for more than six months, says Dr. Friedman. It's also expensive, and fibroids return when treatment ends.

Some physicians express mixed feelings about GnRH. Talk to your own physician.

For Prolapsed Uterus

About 16 percent of hysterectomies (and over 33 percent for women over age 55) are for uterine prolapse, when the uterus drops because of weakening internal supports. In extreme cases, the uterus "falls" outside the vagina.

Kegel exercises can halt or correct mild prolapse. Dr. Hutchins prescribes them, along with estrogen cream or tablets, to firm up the region and says he often sees "substantial improvement."

How do you do a Kegel? Dr. Hutchins tells women that it's best to do them sitting down. "Tighten the muscles around the vagina. Count to ten and release. Do that ten times. Do each exercise three times a day or as often as you can. You may see results in two months."

A pessary may do the trick. This ring-shaped device fits inside the vagina, supporting the uterus and vaginal walls. It can be worn full-time, or just part-time during unusual stress to the uterus, says Dr. Hutchins. "I had a patient in her forties who was an aerobics instructor. When teaching, she would have symptoms of prolapse, a sensation of pelvic pressure. So we fitted her with an inflatable pessary—you insert it deflated and inflate it to the point of comfort. She can jump around as much as she wants and take it out when she's done."

Pessaries must be changed and cleaned frequently, and they can cause inflammation, unpleasant discharge, or ulceration if they're not cleaned regularly or fitted properly.

It may be possible to resuspend the uterus. For severe prolapse, some doctors do surgery to resuspend the uterus in the abdomen, but it's an uncommon surgery that comes with no guarantees. Gravity and stress can bring the uterus back down.

For Unusual Bleeding

Irregular or profuse bleeding is usually related to hormonal fluctuation. But there are many other possible triggers: infections, fibroids, an IUD, and others. Such bleeding is extremely important to investigate—especially in post-menopausal women and women approaching meno-pause—since unusual bleeding can be a symptom of uterine cancer. In younger women, uterine cancer is uncommon.

Again, watchful waiting may be the most prudent course of action. According to gynecologist Herbert Keyser, M.D., author of *Women under the Knife*, "Often (in women under 40) the best treatment is doing nothing but watchful waiting. In my practice I have observed young women whose heavy or irregular menses corrected themselves once the stress in their lives was resolved."

Hormonal treatments may have a positive effect. Birth control pills or progesterone are the most common treatments for heavy bleeding and can create a more normal period or regulate flow. Not all women can tolerate hormone therapy, however.

Endometrial ablation may be another option. If all else fails, a controversial new option is ablation of the endometrium (the uterine lining). A laser or an electrified knife is used to create scar tissue that prevents bleeding. The procedure is done through the vagina, and the patient can go home the same day.

Milton Goldrath, M.D., chief of gynecology at Sinai Hospital in Detroit, developed the procedure using a laser. He says that of 400 patients he's treated, 70 percent are not bleeding at all, and another 30 percent are spotting. Twenty-four women eventually had hysterectomies anyway.

"The problem is, not many surgeons know how to do the procedure, so it's not widely used yet," says Franklin Loffer, M.D., director of gynecologic endoscopy at Maricopa Medical Center in Phoenix, Arizona. Note, too, the procedure carries all the surgical risks of hysterectomy. It should be used only to curb hemorrhagic bleeding, not normally heavy periods. And it cannot be used for women who may wish further pregnancies, as it usually leaves the patient sterile.

If you're considering endometrial ablation, get a second opinion and find a qualified surgeon.

For Endometriosis

Almost 20 percent of hysterectomies are performed for endometriosis. This often painful problem occurs when endometrial tissue—the same kind that's normally inside the uterus—grows outside of the uterus. The "implants" can grow on the outer wall of the uterus or on other body organs like the ovaries, bowels, bladder, or appendix. Endometriosis wanes at menopause, when estrogen levels fall.

Hysterectomy is not a certain solution to endometriosis. It would have to include an oophorectomy, to cut off estrogen. Even that doesn't always work, because a small piece of the ovary can remain in the body, generating estrogen. Posthysterectomy estrogen replacement therapy can bring back endometriosis, too, notes Celso-Ramon Garcia, M.D., director of reproductive surgery at the Hospital of the University of Pennsylvania.

Hormone therapy may bring relief. Birth control pills can deliver a low, controlled amount of estrogen and a potent amount of progesterone, which keeps endometriosis under control. Stronger hormone treatments are sometimes prescribed to temporarily quell the condition until menopause, pregnancy, or surgery. Danazol, a synthetic male hormone, suppresses the ovaries, depriving the body of estrogen and creating false menopause. It often causes undesirable side effects, such as weight gain, depression, and hot flashes. GnRH is used in a similar way, and most women find the side effects more acceptable than those of danazol.

Laser surgery offers a new solution. Conventional surgery involves opening the abdominal cavity and cutting tissue out with a scalpel or cauterizing it. There's also a new, state-of-the-art surgery, performed by a laser-equipped laparoscope through small incisions in the abdomen. Camran Nezhat, M.D., director of the Fertility and Endocrinology Center at the Northside Hospital in Atlanta, Georgia, pioneered the procedure and has received national attention for his success with it. He calls it videolaseroscopy. Because the abdomen is not opened, and because lasers are used (lasers seal off blood vessels as they cut), there is less risk of infection, scarring, bleeding, and pain, and the patient can go home the same day. The procedure appears to be more successful than conventional surgery for severe endometriosis. Once the excess tissue is zapped, it doesn't grow back, although it can appear in other locations.

This technique is not yet widely used, says Dr. Nezhat. "Perhaps 2 percent of doctors who operate on endometriosis are doing it." He also emphasizes the importance of finding an experienced surgeon.

Making Alternatives Work

To explore options other than a hysterectomy, you'll need the best doctor you can find. Seek out a physician certified by the American Board of Obstetrics and Gynecology—preferably, one who is on staff at a teaching hospital or major medical center.

When in doubt about the diagnosis or recommendation, don't hesitate to get a second opinion—or a second diagnostic test. Your best defense against an unnecessary hysterectomy is information. Read books, find people who've had the surgery (or the alternatives), contact support groups, locate the medical literature. And then show them to your doctor, says HERS (Hysterectomy Educational Resources and Services) president Nora W. Coffey. "That's the way to get a doctor's cooperation, and not hostility."

Participate in the decision! This will not only help you avoid a hysterectomy but will also help protect you against depression if you do require one, says Harvard Medical School psychiatrist Malkah Notman, M.D.

For Pelvic Pain

Pelvic pain has many causes. Sometimes it comes from the uterus. But pelvic pain also can originate in the bowel or urinary tract or can stem from a pinched nerve. Pelvic pain should be investigated thoroughly before treatment is begun.

Treat the pain. The University of California, Los Angeles, Pelvic-Pain Management Program was set up four years ago to offer an alternative to hysterectomy, says psychologist Linda Kames, Psy.D., clinical assistant professor in the Department of Anesthesiology at UCLA. "The idea for the program came to me at UCLA's Pain Management Center, where we were getting posthysterectomy patients who were still having pain—pretty much the same pain as they had before the hysterectomy. Hysterectomy is not a good idea if it's done solely for undiagnosed pain."

Like other pain clinics, the program seeks to treat the pain—not the causes—with an interdisciplinary approach, involving gynecologists, anesthesiologists, psychologists, and acupuncturists.

Most of the patients get twice-weekly acupuncture treatments. In psychotherapy, they learn coping skills, such as self-hypnosis and stress avoidance. Some patients are given low doses of antidepressants, which can alleviate pain, says Dr. Kames. Another method used occasionally is the trigger-point injection. (This technique, originally developed for headaches, involves injecting sensitive muscle areas with a local anesthetic.)

Dr. Kames suggests that women experiencing pelvic pain talk to their gynecologist about finding a pain program.

For Incontinence

It's unknown how many hysterectomies are performed for the sole purpose of relieving urinary incontinence, but it is occasionally done, says Neil M. Resnick, M.D., director of the Continence Center at Brigham and Women's Hospital, Boston.

Just say no. In truth, hysterectomy is not considered an appropriate treatment for incontinence except in the very rare instances when the condition is associated with a uterine abnormality. "Incontinence is a symptom, and the cause should be carefully diagnosed before undertaking any surgery," says Dr. Resnick.

CHAPTER 37

New Cures for Impotence

Up to 90 percent of men are suffering needlessly.

The statistic is not likely to come up at the local tavern or next month's meeting of the Lions Club: An estimated 10 million American men are impotent—roughly one in nine. They are unable to obtain and maintain an erection satisfactory for sexual intercourse.

"The real tragedy, though, is that as many as 90 percent of these men may be suffering needlessly," says renowned New York City urologist E. Douglas Whitehead, M.D., director of the Association for Male Sexual Dysfunction in New York City. "Impotence is primarily an epidemic with a cure. Great strides have been made in recent years, not just in diagnosing the causes of impotence but in doing something about them."

Perhaps the greatest of those strides has been the discovery that between 50 and 70 percent of all cases of impotence are physical rather than psychological in origin. "The obtaining of an erection is an immensely complex physiological process involving highly intricate systems—hormonal, neurological, and vascular. A breakdown in any one of these systems can result in erection failure," says Dr. Whitehead.

A man in the gloom of a sexual failure isn't apt to consider that, however. "He's probably going to assume he's suffering from a psychological problem that is going to either go away or require psychological counseling he may not be willing to endure," Dr. Whitehead says. "The end result, either way, is that he's not going to seek treatment. And so the curable plague goes on."

Compounding the problem has been the ignorance of some physicians regarding the new cures for impotence that are now available. "It comes from physicians of the old guard, especially," Dr. Whitehead says. "A man may finally get up the courage to tell his family doctor he's experiencing erection problems, only to hear some cute cliché, such as that all good things must at some point come to an end. What the doctor should be saying is that where there's a will, there's usually a way. If a man has a desire for sex—regardless of his age—the chances are now extremely good that he can have it." Any man told by his family doctor that he's reached the end of his sexual rope shouldn't take no for an answer; he should schedule a detailed physical exam with a urologist, Dr. Whitehead says. "The chances are good that a physical and treatable cause will be found."

And if one is not? "The recommendation then will be for psychological counseling by a sex therapist or a psychiatrist. What men need to realize above all is that sexual dysfunction—just like high blood pressure or being overweight or having high cholesterol—is now a treatable problem. Not until a man invests some time and effort, however, will appropriate treatment be found." That being the case, here are six steps a man faced with impotence should consider.

Step 1:
Beware the Macho Lifestyle

Advertisers would have us believe that booze, tobacco, and life in the fast lane go hand in hand with sex, but in reality these things can keep it from ever getting out of the garage. Sexuality, especially as a man gets older, "is a finely tuned affair and hence quite susceptible to interference from chemical as well as psychological sources," Dr. Whitehead says. "Men must realize that what's bad for physical health tends also to be bad for sexual health." Take the following examples.

Alcohol. Not only can alcohol sabotage potency in the short run, chronic alcohol abuse can blunt the ability of the testicles to produce testosterone, thus jeopardizing potency permanently. Years of heavy drinking also can

damage the liver in a way that "feminizes" the body's use
of what little testosterone the testicles do produce. The
result can be not just impotence but also testicular shrink-
age and noticeable enlargement of the breasts.

Smoking. Smoking can foil sexual potency by contributing to the buildup of plaque in the arteries—the peripheral
arteries like those within the penis, especially. The result
can be blood flow insufficient to fuel the erection process.
In some men, smoking can thwart potency far more immediately, however, by preventing the amount of arterial
dilation needed for erection. Quitting smoking often restores potency in such cases.

Stress. Stress can spoil the erection process physically
as well as psychologically. Just ask yourself how romantic
you feel the next time you're tired or wired. Feeling relaxed
is an important component in the erection process, Dr.
Whitehead says, something that a lot of men forget.

Step 2:
Consider Medical Conditions

The list of medical complications that can confound the
erection process is a long one. It's important to consider
all of them, however, particularly if you come up short on
other possible causes. Having a complete physical is the
best way to find out for sure whether any of these disorders
are bothering you. Here's some of what your doctor should
be looking for:

- Diabetes
- Atherosclerosis and abnormal blood vessel drainage
- Diseases of the erectile tissue of the penis (Peyronie's
  disease and priapism)
- Hormonal abnormalities
- Neurological diseases, such as Parkinson's disease and
  epilepsy
- Kidney and liver disorders
- Pelvic fractures
- Spinal cord injuries
- The effects of surgery (such as prostate, bladder, or
  rectal) on the pelvic area

Step 3:
Try the "Miracles"
of Modern Medicine

If a medical condition is the cause of your problem, do not by any means think you need to throw in the towel. You have at least three major options, depending on the nature of your disorder.

Penile injections. They're best at salvaging potency in cases where dysfunction is due to nerve damage—diabetes, surgery, or spinal cord injury, for example. An injection of a chemical called papaverine (sometimes combined with phentolamine) is self-administered shortly before intercourse, arteries of the penis are caused to dilate, and bingo: an erection that lasts even after ejaculation. There is some risk with the injections, however (permanent damage to the penis if an erection lasts longer than four hours and internal scar buildup are two examples). They are not recommended for use more than twice weekly.

Surgery. Blocked arteries that may be preventing blood from traveling to the penis can sometimes be reopened or bypassed, and leaky veins in the penis that may be preventing erection can be tied off. Perhaps the most dramatic new surgical procedure for restoring potency, however, is the penile implant.

The penile implant. The idea may seem drastic and even macabre, but it can work. Surveys indicate that between 80 and 90 percent of men and their sexual partners report being satisfied with the results of implant surgery, and over 125,000 such operations have been done. Here's an assessment of the basic types of implants currently available, offered by Richard E. Berger, M.D., and Deborah Berger in *BioPotency: A Guide to Sexual Success.*

Semirigid implants can be installed under a local anesthetic, usually on an outpatient basis. The recovery time usually is shorter than with inflatable implants, because the surgery is less elaborate. There is less chance of surgical complications, and there are no mechanical parts that can malfunction. These implants usually are less costly than inflatables.

With *inflatable implants*, the size of the implant—and erection—can be controlled by how much fluid is pumped into it. The erection produced is closer in appearance to what would be produced naturally, and the implant has less chance of changing position within the penis. Inflatable implants are easier for a surgeon to work around if bladder problems develop.

Step 4:
Check the Effects of Medications

Even longer than the list of illnesses that can affect potency is the list of medicines. If you suspect a drug might be the root of your erection woes, check with your doctor about switching to an alternate drug or an alternate treatment. Do not make any changes on your own.

Step 5:
Probe the Mind Factor

Though most causes of impotence are now thought to be primarily physical, the mind also can be a factor. Psychological impotence is more likely than physical impotence to come on suddenly—that's one clue—but you can get a better idea simply by noticing the behavior of your penis at night. If you get nocturnal erections or wake up erect in the morning, your problem is apt to be psychological rather than physical in origin. You could be suffering from simple "performance anxiety" brought on by a past failure, or you could be plagued by something more complicated. In either case, however, sex therapy by a sex therapist or psychotherapy by a psychiatrist may be your answer.

The best candidates for successful sex therapy or psychotherapy? Men who are not afraid to dig deep and who come to therapy strongly motivated, Dr. Berger says.

Step 6:
Take Care of Yourself

Perhaps the most encouraging news to emerge from what scientists now know about sexual potency, however, is simply that it's mostly under your control. "Sexual desire needs a healthy body to put it to work," Dr. Whitehead says. "Few men realize that the same behaviors that can clog the arteries of the heart also can clog the arteries of the penis. This makes proper diet and regular exercise important components of keeping sexually fit."

High serum cholesterol levels, a high percentage of body fat, high blood pressure—all are controllable and all have been shown to contribute to the risk of potency breakdown. If you want to prolong your potency, try to follow these essential guidelines:

- Eat a low-cholesterol, low-fat, high-fiber diet. Maintain your proper weight.
- Keep your blood pressure at a normal measurement.
- Exercise regularly.
- Don't smoke, chew, or sniff tobacco.
- Drink alcohol in moderation only.

CHAPTER 38

Update on Minoxidil, the Hair Saver

It's not the miracle drug you may have hoped for. But many will bless it anyway.

Baldness has always been a hair-raising experience for men, a self-questioning mind game pitting oneself against the inevitable. From questionable snake oil remedies to laughable cheap toupees, millions of balding men have long gone to great lengths to hide the bald truth about themselves.

Then along came minoxidil, viewed by many as an answer to "the great recession" suffered by 55 million American men. Its maker, the Upjohn Company, stands to see earnings increased by 36 percent for each million men who try minoxidil for a year. The pharmaceutical firm felt those profits were worth the gamble of having a multi-million-dollar production plant ready well in advance of approval from the Food and Drug Administration (FDA), which came in August of 1988, after two years of waiting.

But corporate gains from minoxidil—Rogaine Topical Solution, as it's known by prescription at pharmacies nationwide—may be more impressive than the results it has on waning manes.

"The truth about this drug is that it will turn out to be great for some men but a huge disappointment for others," says Harry L. Roth, M.D., a clinical professor of dermatology at the University of California, San Francisco, and the director of one of the 27 separate year-long studies (involving 2,300 men) which were responsible for earning minoxidil its FDA approval. "It's important that men be forewarned of what minoxidil can and can't do, and for whom. Men who are older than 35 whose baldness is quite extensive will not do well. The drug is most effective for men in their early twenties and thirties whose hair loss has started only within the past several years and is not advanced."

Adds Elise Olsen, M.D., an assistant professor of medicine at the Duke University Medical Center, who also directed an FDA minoxidil test: "Men who have bald areas on the tops of their heads measuring two inches in diameter or less are the ones who will do best with this drug. I would be reluctant to prescribe it for men whose conditions are considerably more advanced than that, unless their goal would be just to slow their hair loss down."

Better as a Defense Than a Cure

Although minoxidil may not turn out to be the great baldness buster hoped for when its hair-raising powers were accidentally discovered 15 years ago (the drug is traditionally for blood pressure control), the stuff stands a good chance of at least being able to call itself a hair *saver*. Even men in test studies who saw no actual growth felt that minoxidil at least *slowed* hair loss.

"The drug is clearly better for retarding hair loss than for growing new hair," says Gene T. Izuno, M.D., dermatologist at the Scripps Clinic in La Jolla, California, where another of the FDA's minoxidil trials was conducted. Adds Dominic Brandy, M.D., medical director of the Cosmetic Hair Replacement Surgery Center in Pittsburgh: "I will be prescribing minoxidil more as a defense against baldness than as a cure for it."

The Bald Truths

But some die-hard chrome domes are willing to gamble the $700 a year it costs to use minoxidil for a head of hair. Before throwing away their money (or setting themselves up for disappointment), they should know some minoxidil facts:

- It works best on men younger than 30 whose hair loss is not extensive and has started only recently, preferably within the last five years. Even among these prime candidates, only a third can expect good results (at least a doubling in hair density), while about 40 percent can expect fair results (hair thickness will double and the bald spot will shrink, but not disappear). The others will experience virtually no change, though they may experience a retarding of hair loss.
- Minoxidil cannot grow new hair where there is none, but rather can only thicken and lengthen existing hairs, thin and tiny (vellus) though they may be. It also doesn't grow hair at the temples or forehead; it works best on bald spots on the top of the head measuring two inches in diameter or less.
- It must be applied twice daily for at least four to six months—and sometimes a full year—before *any* results are seen. And because it is a lifetime commitment, a man who stops using it will lose whatever hair he has gained within about six months.
- Minoxidil has been shown to be effective for male pattern baldness only. Studies are currently in progress testing its effectiveness on female pattern baldness and alopecia areata—sudden hair loss due to illness or stress.

- It is relatively free of side effects (slight scalp irritation being the only reported one), although there is some fear that, as a high blood pressure medication, it could cause complications for men with cardiovascular problems. Be sure to check with your physician and get regular checkups once you start using minoxidil if you fall into this group.

The Alternatives

There are, of course, other treatments and procedures available for balding or thinning hair. Here's a summary of some of them.

The hair lift. Most recent and dramatic of the surgical alternatives is the hair lift. In a series of three or four operations, bald scalp is removed and scalp with hair is moved from the back and sides of the head to the top of the head. Results can be remarkable, but depending on how many operations are needed, cost ranges from $3,000 to $15,000.

Scalp reduction. Scalp reduction removes a section of bald scalp from the top of the head. Then the sides are drawn upward to minimize the size of the bald area. This procedure is used when the bald spot is not large enough to warrant a full hair lift. Several operations can be performed a few months apart, the result being a reduction in the bald area. For men whose scalps are tight, inflatable balloons may be inserted beneath the scalp several weeks before surgery, to give the scalp a stretch. The cost ranges from $500 to $2,000 per operation.

Hair transplant. Practiced for more than 30 years, this procedure entails taking plugs of hair from the back and sides of the head and surgically embedding them where hair is lacking. Plugs can vary in size from fairly large (8 to 20 hairs) to very small, some consisting of a single hair. Bad hair transplants are a very common problem. Prices range between $10 and $40 a plug, with a complete job costing about $6,000, depending on how many plugs are required.

Hair weaving. The procedure is not surgical but merely cosmetic in that it attaches extensions, either natural or synthetic, to existing hairs. On the down side, every four to six weeks (as the hair grows out), the extensions must be repositioned.

The hairpiece. For between $600 and $2,000, you can get a custom-made piece that perfectly matches your existing hair. Most toupees last only about a year or two, but a man should always have at least two. With the $20-a-month fees for servicing and cleaning by a professional, figure that 30 years of toupee use will cost about $85,200, says Paul Kochanasz, a hairpiece specialist in Allentown, Pennsylvania. (Self-service will cost about half as much.)

Synthetic pieces are better for active, sports-minded men because they hold up to weather and water better and are easier to keep clean. Natural pieces do tend to look slightly better at first, but the harsh processing done to Oriental hair—the largest hair source—makes the hair break down sooner. Costwise, figure about $150 more for a natural than a synthetic piece in the $1,000 category.

PART VIII: MEDICAL
ADVANCES FOR A MORE
BEAUTIFUL YOU

Flash Reports

DENTAL IMPLANT UPDATE

Do you have an artificial tooth, a bridge, or dentures? If so, you know the inconvenience, embarrassment, even the pain of having your false teeth betray you at the worst moment. Avoiding all this is what's so appealing about "permanent" teeth, or dental implants.

Dental implants are metal posts set into holes drilled into the jawbone (just as you'd set screws into a piece of wood) and capped by artificial teeth. The teeth are screwed or glued onto the posts, which extend above the gum line.

Dental implants have actually been marketed for about 20 years, but only within the last 10 years have materials and techniques improved to where they are a reasonable option. Still, many questions about how different implants might work in different patients need to be answered. Only one manufacturer, Nobelpharma (Branemark) of Sweden, has obtained American Dental Association (ADA) approval, though other manufacturers may receive approval soon. Manufacturers' studies suggest that in good candidates—people with strong jawbones and no infections—implants can last 20 years or more. Realistically, though, there is no guarantee of how long any implant may last.

How do you get a good implant? "It's very important to choose a qualified dentist, usually an oral surgeon or periodontist, for this procedure," says Max Listgarten,

D.D.S., of the University of Pennsylvania School of Dental Medicine and a member of the National Institutes of Health review panel on dental implants.

Unfortunately, finding a dentist qualified to do implants may be difficult. Because implant dentistry is a new field with no set criteria for recognizing a bona fide implant specialist, the ADA has not yet agreed to recognize implant dentistry as a specialty. Some boards to which a dentist may belong have no qualifying criteria for membership.

"Contact your local dental society," Dr. Listgarten says. "Find out where the doctor was trained, and for how long. And talk with other dentists before making a choice." Since implants run about $1,000 a tooth, you'll want to be sure of what you're getting!

DON'T LET YOUR DRUGS BURN YOU

Have you ever gotten a sunburn so fast you thought you were standing under a hole in the ozone layer? In fact, it's more likely the result of something you're taking—or wearing. Some diuretics, diabetes drugs, antibiotics like tetracycline, and sulfa drugs can cause sun sensitivity. So can oral contraceptives, the acne medicine Accutane, and fragrances such as lime, musk, sandalwood, and cedar. Even some sunscreens contain ingredients that can make you burn. Takers and wearers beware!

CHEW YOUR TEETH WHITER

Researchers may have found a new role for sugarless gum made with xylitol, a natural sweetener found in fruits and vegetables.

In a recent study at the University of Michigan School of Dentistry, 28 students were divided into three groups. One group chewed ten pieces of xylitol gum daily for two weeks. Another group chewed gum sweetened with a combination of xylitol and sorbitol (another nonsugar sweetener). The third group chewed gum sweetened with sorbitol alone.

Plaque was significantly reduced in the xylitol and xylitol-sorbitol groups, while it actually increased in the sorbitol users.

By interfering with the growth of microorganisms that form plaque, xylitol makes cavity-promoting plaque looser and easier to remove with brushing, says Kauko Makinen, Ph.D., who conducted the study.

In fact, in a previous study by Dr. Makinen, cavity-prone children reduced cavities by up to 80 percent with the use of xylitol gum.

What's more, a recent study by researchers at the University of Turku, in Finland, found that gum sweetened with xylitol reduced cavities in children *even after they stopped using it.*

In the study, 172 children who chewed the gum two or three times a day for two to three years averaged 53 percent fewer cavities than 152 kids who didn't. Three years after they stopped chewing, the xylitol chompers still had 51 percent fewer cavities.

CHAPTER 39

Are You Right for Liposuction?

Ironically, the procedure that can successfully suck out fatty bulges is not for the obese.

Suction-assisted lipectomy—commonly called liposuction or lipoplasty—is a procedure that permanently removes deposits of excess fat that can't be removed by diet and exercise.

"A promising candidate for liposuction is someone of normal weight, or only minimally overweight, who is disproportionately heavy in certain areas, such as thighs, hips, or waist," says Andrew Ordon, M.D., a New York City plastic surgeon. "It can be disheartening if you're doing everything right—watching what you eat, getting plenty of exercise—and you still have 'love handles' or 'saddlebags.' "

One of the more appealing aspects of the procedure is that it permanently recontours your body. "After you reach adulthood, the number of fat cells you have is fixed," explains Dr. Ordon. "When we remove them, they won't regrow, but the size of the remaining cells can vary according to diet and exercise. If you do gain weight after liposuction, you'll gain all over—you won't have disproportionate bulges."

Still, the whole idea of instant eradication of bulges that heaven and earth can't move is so attractive that surgeons have to keep reminding people of liposuction's limits.

First, they say, liposuction is not for the obese. Says Dr. Ordon, "If you are significantly overweight, you're a poor candidate for liposuction alone, because there's a limit to how much fat can safely or effectively be suctioned off." Four to six pounds is about the top limit, which wouldn't do much for someone far above his or her ideal weight.

Second, the operation is only for those in good health.

Third, it can be successful only on people with resilient skin. Resilience ensures that after the fat has been surgically extracted, the skin will re-form over the new contours and won't hang like a deflated balloon. And the best indicator of resilience, say plastic surgeons, is not your chronological age but your skin's "physiological age." Most people who fit the bill, however, are in their forties or younger.

Fourth, even if your skin is perfect, it's possible that some unevenness or rippling will show. Newer and smaller instruments in the hands of an experienced surgeon, however, dramatically reduce the chances of this.

Fifth, liposuction can't do anything about cellulite.

Liposuction can be performed in a hospital or an outpatient facility, depending on what the patient and surgeon determine is best.

How It's Done

The patient is given either a local anesthetic, which numbs the area to be treated, or general anesthesia. The surgeon then makes a small incision and inserts a blunt-ended instrument called a cannula—it looks like a metal soda straw—through the skin into the layer of fat below. At the other end of the cannula, a suction unit is attached. Using the cannula, the surgeon dislodges fat, and the suction unit extracts it. The incision is then closed. When it heals, a small scar remains. All this may sound easy, but it's not. The skill and technique of the surgeon can make the difference between good results and unevenness or rippled skin.

After the operation, the liposuctioned area is compressed tightly, either with elastic gauze or a long surgical girdle. This dressing helps the skin conform with the new body contours and helps reduce temporary swelling and bruising that are common effects of this surgery. Depending on how much fat was removed and how well you heal, you can expect to wear a dressing from three weeks to three months.

The amount of pain or discomfort after surgery is moderate and varies from individual to individual. "The worst period is within four to five days after surgery," says Dr. Ordon. "Localized numbness or discomfort may be experienced for a longer period of time."

Generally, healing is slower the older you are. Conditions like high blood pressure, smoking, or diabetes are factors that lessen the chances of good, quick healing.

"You will see approximately 70 percent of your final result within three weeks of surgery," says Dr. Ordon. "But the final 100 percent result you may not see for three months."

An Informed Choice

Liposuction is elective surgery that, like any surgery, involves a certain amount of risk. But the risk is comparatively low. Liposuction has a morbidity (complication) rate that is lower than that of tonsillectomy. The mortality rate is also extremely low—1 death in 10,000 operations.

"Although liposuction is safe and effective when done properly, there are several factors that increase the risks or call for special care," says plastic surgeon Simon Fredricks, M.D., who was chairman of the American Society of Plastic and Reconstructive Surgeons' committee to research liposuction. "These include the use of the technique in conjunction with other body-sculpting procedures, removal of too much fat (which can, among other things, create deformities), and inadequate physician training or facilities. Some body contour problems are best solved by using liposuction with other plastic surgery techniques. But it's vital that such operations be performed by professionals who are experienced body contour surgeons."

Finding the right surgeon requires some careful screening on the part of the patient. "Unfortunately, anyone with an M.D., regardless of his or her level of training or experience, can put an ad in the paper saying they can perform liposuction," says Dr. Fredricks. "Or they can take a weekend course in liposuction and get a certificate to hang on the office wall."

So to be safe and to be sure that the doctor is properly trained, people should go to a surgeon who is certified by the American Board of Plastic Surgery and who has had additional training and experience in suction-assisted lipectomy. To verify that a physician is qualified to perform liposuctions, call the board, toll free, at 1-800-635-0635.

"Don't be shy about asking your prospective surgeon what his training is," Dr. Fredricks says, "or how much additional experience he has in this procedure. He should not be offended if you ask him how many he has done. You're entitled to that information."

Finally, it's vital to be honest with both your doctor and yourself about your reasons for this surgery. You have to remember that liposuction is not a substitute for exercise and proper diet.

CHAPTER 40

Reduce Wrinkles
with Retin-A

Dermatologists are still enthusiastic but add some precautions for users of this wonder drug.

Several years ago, a scientist discovered a new and exciting use for an old topical anti-acne medication—repairing wrinkles in sun-damaged skin. The medication's brand name was Retin-A, and the scientist was Albert Kligman, M.D., professor of dermatology. Most people had never heard of either one. But today they're both famous. Retin-A has now been shown to improve the skin's appearance by reducing wrinkles, eliminating freckles (especially when used in conjunction with hydroquinone), and regressing solar keratoses (skin blotches that can become malignant). Studies are now being conducted worldwide on Retin-A's benefits. And Dr. Kligman gets credit for starting it all.

So these days lots of people want to use Retin-A to banish wrinkles. But is it right for you? Here's Dr. Kligman's list of factors to consider if you're thinking of using Retin-A.

Side Effects

"Irritation is the only negative side effect I've seen in 17 years of working with Retin-A," says Dr. Kligman, director of the Clinic for Aging Skin and professor of dermatology at the University of Pennsylvania School of Medicine. "And an experienced dermatologist should have at least some clues to what kind of a reaction you will have. For instance, if you're someone who blushes easily, you're more likely to have a strong reaction.

"I think a lot of irritation is preventable by giving the

patient full counseling on the proper use of Retin-A. I don't start a patient on a Retin-A program with less than a 25-minute consultation."

Barbara Gilchrest, M.D., professor and chairperson of dermatology at Boston University School of Medicine, thinks that the initial irritation may be unacceptable to some people.

"People should be advised," says Dr. Gilchrest, also a senior scientist at the U.S. Department of Agriculture's Human Nutrition Research Center on Aging at Tufts University, "that they might have a period of weeks to several months when they'll have some difficulty with their skin that they hadn't had before. Your skin will peel and be easily irritated, and may be red and blotchy. For most people, it's a fairly minor reaction that lasts for only a few weeks."

Other Factors

You also have to realize that Retin-A is for life. When you stop using it, your skin goes back to where it was before treatment.

You start by using Retin-A nightly. When you've achieved maximum benefit—and this varies from person to person—you can cut down to a maintenance program of three to five times a week. But this requires a real commitment to using Retin-A.

"An exciting point, however," says Jonathan A. Weiss, M.D., assistant professor of dermatology at Emory University Medical School and Clinic, "is that when you start using Retin-A, the improvement continues and becomes more impressive with time for up to a year or more."

Another consideration is that if you use Retin-A, you have to apply a sunscreen with a sun protection factor of at least 15 every time you go outside. "If you're not willing to use sunscreens and other sun protection," says Dr. Gilchrest, "you shouldn't even consider Retin-A. Not only doesn't it make any sense to try to prevent a problem that you're causing at the same time, but Retin-A itself is a sun sensitizer." This means that if you use it and go outside without sun protection, you're more likely than normal to get a bad sunburn, especially in the early weeks of therapy.

Another possible concern: After using Retin-A, you may not feel that the difference in your appearance is dramatic enough. "It depends in part on how damaged your skin is to begin with and how much this damage bothers you," says Dr. Weiss. "Our data have shown that you can get measurable improvement in people with both severe and mild sun damage. But the less sun damage you have, the more subtle and less noticeable the results of Retin-A will be."

Retin-A Rip-Offs

One of the negative results of the continuing excitement about Retin-A has been a host of companies trying to cash in on the recognition that's being given to Retin-A.

The medication is a patented derivative of a vitamin A compound that contains retinoic acid. Several companies advertise products with ingredients whose names sound like Retin-A and that are, in fact, chemically related: retinyl or retinol. And they imply the results of their products will be the same as those of Retin-A.

It is a prescription drug only, approved by the Food and Drug Administration (FDA) at this time for the treatment of acne, not for anti-aging. It's perfectly fine for a qualified physician who's familiar with the studies and the drug itself to treat wrinkles with Retin-A. But it's not a treatment you can order by mail.

Advertisements for these sound-alike products started appearing all over the country and even in Mexico. It's just about impossible for the FDA to keep ahead of these fly-by-night companies, so it's a case of "consumer, beware."

Some of the investigations that were undertaken by the FDA to prevent misuse of Retin-A were of clinics that were creating products under their own labels. In those cases some of the products did contain the active ingredient retinoic acid. The problem here was that Retin-A is not a very stable ingredient, and there was no way of checking how carefully and accurately the products were being made.

Ortho, the drug company that makes Retin-A, spends

millions of dollars so the consumer can be certain that the 0.01 percent Retin-A cream your doctor prescribes contains exactly 0.01 percent active retinoic acid. "Without knowing how much retinoic acid is active in the product, you cannot say whether the product is useful, useless, or even dangerous," warns Faye Peterson of the FDA's Office of Public Affairs.

If you're interested in Retin-A, get off to the right start. Consult a dermatologist who has experience with it. He or she should be able to answer your questions and give you a thorough explanation of how to use Retin-A. Look for someone who will be available to answer any questions you may have.

CHAPTER 41

Battling Blemishes

Sunlight won't help. Neither will scrubs. Here's a routine that will.

Acne has never been strictly a teenage blight. But most people feel that they're unusual if they're past 30 and still battling blemishes. Unusual they're not.

"We're seeing an increased number of adult women with acne," says Alan R. Shalita, M.D., chairman of the Department of Dermatology at Downstate Medical Center, State University of New York. "We don't know if there's actually more acne. We do know that more women than ever have careers, and it's embarrassing to have pimples. We hope that they may be more aware that there's now good treatment available."

Why Me? Why Now?

Hormones are factors in acne for both teens and adults, because they can stimulate the oil glands in your skin to secrete more oil. When you're a teenager, it's puberty that brings on swings in hormone levels and the resulting blemishes. But in your twenties, thirties, and up, you may produce an increased amount of male hormones, which can cause your skin to break out.

"Some blemishes may get worse because of efforts to hide them," says Dr. Shalita. "People develop a couple of pimples on their chin and cover them up during a meeting or luncheon by resting their chin in their hand. What happens is that the heat and friction just aggravate their acne."

Many adults who know that sunbathing isn't good for the skin's general health believe that sunlight is beneficial to their acne. "Sunlight is more likely to be a cause of acne than it is a cure," Dr. Shalita says. "Baking in the sun may not only worsen acne, it can also make certain ingredients in cosmetics and skin care products acnegenic [cause blemishes]."

The Maybes

Dietary causes of acne have yet to be scientifically proven. "As a matter of fact," says Dr. Shalita, "there have been formal studies where people were given chocolate or dairy products and then were compared with a control group. In each study there was no significant difference between the two groups."

Stress is another "maybe" in acne causes. There are no well-documented studies that implicate stress as a cause of acne. "After all, it would be hard to get a group of people to be willingly so stressed that we could determine whether stress makes their skin break out," Dr. Shalita says. But there's plenty of anecdotal evidence linking stress to acne. "Just from my own clinical observations, I'd say there is a connection between the two."

Acne Skin Care

Acne is a chronic condition. This means you have to follow a regular program of preventive maintenance to loosen oil plugs and acne-causing bacteria that clog your pores, and then keep the pores as clean as possible.

Be careful how you go about it, however. The bacteria causing the problem are not surface bacteria. Harsh scrubbing to clear out pores can irritate your skin and make the condition worse. "Use a soft washcloth or your hands. I feel that scrubs and abrasive sponges do more harm than good for people with acne," says Dr. Shalita.

If you're under treatment for your acne, be sure your cleanser is very mild, because the medication you're using to clear up your blemishes is probably already drying up your complexion. "I recommend a mild soap, like Dove, Purpose, or Neutrogena, and washing only twice a day. That's enough for most adult skin," Dr. Shalita advises. "Your doctor may also recommend a cleanser that contains salicylic acid. This will loosen the plugs of debris relatively gently, allowing you to wash them away."

After your skin is clean, you want to discourage new blemishes from forming and limit the severity of pimples if they do form. "Antibacterial lotions with benzoyl peroxide are excellent products for this purpose. They can be bought without a prescription. They will, however, cause a skin irritation in some people, so be sure to follow the manufacturer's instructions carefully. If your skin becomes excessively dry or red, try using them less often or discontinue use entirely. There are also cover-ups that hide blemishes while they work to dry them up.

"The mistake that some people make is to just dab these anti-acne preparations on the individual pimples," Dr. Shalita says. "If you have acne, you should ideally be using these products to prevent new pimples by spreading the treatment all over the area that's involved."

Acne, associated in teen years with oily skin, can easily exist side by side with normal to dry skin as you mature. A common concern for adults with acne is that most acne treatments are drying for already dry skin. This need not be a problem, however. "Once you're under treatment, there's no reason you can't use a good moisturizer," states Dr. Shalita. "You should be able to work with your dermatologist to find a moisturizer that won't aggravate your skin.

"Also, all cosmetics are not the villains they were once thought to be. There is some acne that is aggravated by overuse of cosmetics, but such excess is not a major cause."

Blackheads

Blackheads, plugs of oil that fill a pore and darken on contact with air, are one of the most noticeable and distressing signs of acne. They are not a sign of uncleanliness, and scrubbing only makes a bad situation worse. They will go away under treatment, but if you can't stand them one minute longer, you can remove them with a blackhead remover. Never use your fingers: You stand a good chance of damaging the skin and leaving scars or infection.

"Blackhead extractors are okay if you use them with the advice and instruction of your dermatologist," says Dr. Shalita. "No matter how you remove the blackheads, however, they'll be back in a month. But by using the extractor, you can look better while your dermatologist attacks the problem on a more permanent basis. Also, if you're on a treatment program that includes topical tretinoin, or Retin-A, blackheads will be much softer and easier to remove.

"If your skin problem worsens," says Dr. Shalita, "and if you see no relief after a couple of months, or if you're concerned about your complexion for any reason, always consult your dermatologist."

An Arsenal of Hope

Today's dermatologist has many weapons in the anti-acne arsenal. Depending on the severity of the problem, your doctor may recommend anything from an over-the-counter preparation to topical prescription treatments like vitamin A acid, or tretinoin (which works to unblock the pores) used in combination with a topical antibacterial or antibiotic.

Patients who don't respond satisfactorily to topical treatments can be put on oral antibiotics and/or low doses of cortisone. "For very severe acne, we increase the dose," says Dr. Shalita. "For the most severe cases, we can prescribe an oral form of the drug Accutane. There are, however, possible side effects with Accutane. And it does cause birth defects, so you must not use the medication while pregnant and should not start treatment until after the first normal menstrual period following a negative pregnancy test. Accutane is also contraindicated for some diabetics. If you have a high level of blood lipids or blood fats, have dry eyes, or wear contacts, your doctor should monitor you more carefully."

A topical form of Accutane is currently being studied. But even though it shows promise, it will be another helpful tool—not a cure.

CHAPTER 42

New, Beautiful Looks in Dentistry

Lengthening teeth with perfectly matched veneers can make you look years younger.

Perfect teeth, white teeth, a movie star's teeth—these are the popular products of cosmetic dentistry. But nowadays cosmetic dentists are doing more than beautifying teeth— they're helping to save them, too. Techniques for repairing, replacing, or whitening teeth are also helping dentists avoid pulling teeth or grinding them way down to make way for improvements. Here's a rundown on some of these breakthroughs that are helping to keep America smiling.

State-of-the-Art Fillings

The right filling can save a tooth, not just because it plugs a hole and puts decay on hold, but also because it makes the tooth less likely to crack over the years. The new composite resin fillings do both and can match your natural tooth color, to boot. Because they stick to a tooth's surface, they require less drilling than metal fillings. And less drilling means less chance that your tooth will split or break over the long haul.

Composite resin fillings have other advantages, too. Since they adhere readily to teeth, they're the preferred material for filling shallow surface cavities. And they insulate sensitive teeth from extreme temperatures. Metal fillings can aggravate sensitive teeth by conducting heat and cold. Installation is relatively painless; no anesthesia is required. Ronald E. Goldstein, D.D.S., clinical professor of restorative dentistry at the Medical College of Georgia, says that to install composite resin fillings correctly takes up to one hour longer per tooth than silver fillings. Resin fillings usually last five to eight years, he says, about the same as the useful life expectancy of silver fillings. Gold fillings, however, may last a lifetime.

The cost of resin fillings is $65 to $450 per tooth (depending on size and other factors), a little more than silver fillings and about one-half to one-third the price of gold fillings.

Porcelain Laminates

Perhaps the most exciting work in dentistry these days is being done with porcelain veneers, or laminates. (No, not the teacup kind of porcelain that chips so easily.) Dentists custom-make the thin laminates to fit onto your teeth—like wood veneers on fine furniture—and use a type of plastic "glue" to bond the laminates to tooth surfaces. The technique can turn broken or cracked teeth into nearly perfect specimens. And it does so without grinding down the existing tooth to a stub (as it would be if a traditional cap were installed).

Laminates are also used on another problem: short teeth. "Some people have teeth that are naturally not as long as the others, and sometimes teeth wear down over the years," says Irwin Smigel, D.D.S., president of the American Society for Dental Aesthetics. "Laminates are perfect for adding the necessary length. One easy way to make older people look younger is to bring their teeth back to the length they were before."

Although porcelain laminates in one form or another have been around since the early part of this century (Shirley Temple had temporary veneers put on for the camera in the 1930s), they've only recently been perfected for general use. The veneers are an outgrowth of composite bonding, which was the dental breakthrough of the 1970s. With bonding, the dentist sculpts a layer, or composite, of plastics directly onto the tooth, where it is "cured" with a hand-held light to form a new tooth "facade." If done right, the bonding looks natural and should last ten years or more if cared for properly. Bonding is still a useful technique for minor chips. But porcelain laminates have three big advantages over bonding. "First, unlike bonding, porcelain laminates have very small odds of chipping once they're in place," says Dr. Smigel. "Second, the laminates are made in a lab by technicians, not in your mouth by the dentist, and baked in an oven before they're installed, not cured in your mouth with lights, as in bonding. So the laminates can be made with greater precision. We can look at the laminates carefully before we put them in your mouth. And if there are any rough spots that might stain over time, we can smooth them down. Third, the porcelain won't discolor as bonding sometimes does. It keeps its color magnificently."

So how does a dentist apply laminates to your teeth? During your first visit, he or she prepares the teeth by grinding off a paper-thin layer of enamel (about ½ millimeter), then takes an impression of the teeth by coating them with a pastelike material that hardens and then is easily removed. The dentist decides what color the laminates should be (they're available in a whole spectrum of shades), then sends the impression to the lab, which uses it to make the laminates. This first visit could take up to two hours. Your second visit is an audition, where the dentist tries the laminates to make sure they fit. You can preview how the veneers look and how their color matches your other teeth. If something is wrong, the dentist can fix it before the third visit, when the veneers are actually installed. Installation could take as long as three hours for lots of teeth.

All three steps are relatively painless. And important. "These steps shouldn't be rushed," says John R. Calamia, D.D.S., of New York University's Dental School. "The teeth must be well prepped. The work is meticulous.

"The second step, or try-in, is especially crucial. It takes only a few minutes, but it's worth it." Dr. Calamia suggests that you bring a valued friend or relative along on this visit to give an opinion on your new appearance. Dr. Calamia usually does his laminate work in three visits and recommends that you be suspicious of any dentist who doesn't allow for a try-in visit.

The cost of porcelain laminates is from $350 to $900 per tooth.

Resin-Bonded Bridges

Bridges have always been an alternative to giving up on remaining teeth and getting dentures. But now there's a new class of fixed bridges that's a tooth saver in another way. Unlike traditional fixed bridges, these don't require adjacent teeth to be ground down to make room for crowns. They're called resin-bonded fixed bridges, and they get extra points for attractiveness (the metal is hard to see or nonexistent in the newest types) and ease of installation.

With traditional fixed bridges, two new crowns had to be constructed so the bridge could be firmly attached to solid supports. That's a lot of work. But resin-bonded bridges have "wings" that are "glued" with composite bonding directly to etched metal brackets on the two existing adjacent teeth. No grinding and no caps needed. The result is a fixed bridge that costs from one-third to one-half as much as the traditional type. The process takes about 1½ hours, and the bridges may last 5 to 15 years, some dentists say.

One drawback is that these new bridges don't always match adjacent teeth as well as they should. If the adjacent teeth look good, the bridge will blend right in because it looks good, too. But if the adjacent teeth look bad, the bridge will stick out like a sore thumb. In this case, a traditional bridge might be worth the extra expense.

How to Find a Good Cosmetic Dentist

Deciding on a cosmetic dentist is like choosing any doctor; you should take the time to shop around for one who is experienced and can best meet your needs.

- Call or write one of the following for a referral: your local or state dental association; the department of aesthetic dentistry at a university dental school; the American Academy of Esthetic Dentistry, 211 East Chicago Avenue, Suite 948, Chicago, IL 60611; the American Society for Dental Aesthetics, 635 Madison Avenue, New York, NY 10022.
- Ask a friend who's had cosmetic dental work done to give you a referral.
- Quiz the prospective dentist. Ask how long he or she has been doing cosmetic dentistry. (Several years is the right answer.) Ask if he or she keeps up with changes in the field by going to seminars on the latest techniques. Ask to see before-and-after photographs of his or her work.

Another drawback is that the metal brackets on the back side of the adjacent teeth can change the color of thin teeth by blocking the passage of light through the teeth. This isn't a problem with thicker teeth. And dentists have developed a solution for some of these cases. Sometimes the replacement tooth can be attached to tooth-colored porcelain—not metal brackets—on the back of the adjacent teeth.

"I consider this use of porcelain to be experimental," Dr. Goldstein says. "I use them only on people who aren't likely to overstress the porcelain bonds—people who don't grind their teeth or have heavy musculature."

The cost for a resin-bonded fixed bridge is $300 to $1,500 per tooth.

Implants

In times past, if you were missing many teeth and you didn't have enough surrounding teeth to anchor a bridge or partial denture, you had the remaining teeth pulled and got full dentures. But now there may be a way around this predicament: dental implants. They're permanent false teeth that dentists embed right into the jawbone.

"With a person who is missing most of his back teeth, we don't have a way to put a fixed bridge in, because there's nothing to anchor to," says Dr. Calamia. "You can't have a whole string of false teeth hanging in the air, just held on by a few front teeth. Now you can put one or two implants in the back as support for a bridge connecting to the remaining front teeth."

But implants are a big job. The procedure takes several lengthy office visits, plus a waiting period of many weeks to see if the implants "take." It's serious surgery requiring anesthesia. And implants aren't for everyone. If gum disease has eaten away too much jawbone, an implant may not stay in place. And implants require meticulous cleaning and vigilant oral hygiene. "There's still a lot of research needed to determine how well implants work and how long they'll last," says a spokesperson for the American Dental Association. "Techniques are improving. You're definitely going to see a lot more implants to replace single teeth and, farther in the future, even full-mouth implants."

The cost is at least $1,000 per tooth.

Index

A

Ablation of endometrium, 249, 256
Absorption
of drugs, 41, 43, 46, 130
of nutrients, 172
of Vitamin B_{12}, 190
Accutane, 271, 282–83
Acetaminophen, 45, 127, 200
Achilles tendon, 235
Acne, 279–83
Retin-A for, 278, 282
Acne rosacea, 63
Acoustic neuroma, 16–17
Acupuncture, 78, 259
Aging
dry eyes during, 62
and gallstone development, 37
and urinary incontinence, 47, 49
Agoraphobia, 153, 156
AIDS, 68, 140
Alcohol, 172, 182, 265
abuse of, 150
and allergies, 214
as cause of snoring, 226
impotence from, 261–62
and interaction with drugs, 147
and sinusitis, 74
tranquilizing effect of, 145
and urinary tract infection, 78
Alcoholism, 134, 140, 151, 182
Allergies, 16, 72, 177, 212–23, 240
Alopecia areata, 267
Alprazolam, 148, 157
Alzheimer's disease, 133–40
Amcill, 42, 45
Ampicillin, 42, 45

Amputation, 55, 57, 94
Ancanthamoeba keratitis, 197
Anemia, 111–12, 140, 190, 248
Angina, 3, 9
Angioplasty
balloon, 6–8, 9, 10, 23
devices for, 25
for intermittent claudication, 60
laser-assisted, 8, 9
Ankylosing spondylitis, 32
Anorexia, 179
Antibiotic ointment, 201–2
Antibiotics, 271
for acne, 282
for blepharitis, 66
broad-spectrum, 42
and interaction with food, 42
for sinusitis, 74
after sinus surgery, 75
for urinary tract infections, 76
Antibodies
monoclonal, 95–96, 107, 176
radio-labeled, 111
for tumor detection, 89
Anticoagulants, interaction of, with food, 43–44
Antidepressants, 44, 63, 128, 131, 157, 259
Antihistamines, 63, 74, 219, 227
nonsedating, 239–43
Anxiety, 154, 155. *See also* Panic attacks; Stress before medical tests, 183–89
Apnea, sleep, 225–26, 227, 228
Arch supports, 235–36, 238
Argon laser, 11–12, 13, 14, 15
Arterial plaque. *See* Plaque, arterial

Arthritis, 200, 206
  drugs for, 32, 46
  rheumatoid, 32, 64, 134
  spinal, 207, 210
Artificial sweeteners, 172
Artificial tears, 64–65, 68
Aspirin, 45, 46, 200–201
  for gallstone prevention, 37
  for heart attack treatment,
    33
  for heart disease, 59
  for intermittent claudication,
    59
  for migraines, 127
  for stroke dementia, 125–26
Assertiveness training, 156
Asthma, 143, 217–18, 219–20
Atherosclerosis, 2, 19, 20, 21, 22,
    55, 57, 58, 262
Athlete's foot, 201
Autoimmune diseases, 64
Autoimmune hypothesis and
    Alzheimer's disease,
    134–35

B
Back pain, 205–12
Baldness, 265–69
Balloon angioplasty. See
    Angioplasty, balloon
Balloon catheterization, 34
Balloons for plugging ulcers, 1
Barbiturates, 147, 148
Baths, hot, 146–47, 185
Behavioral therapy, 50–52, 129
Bell's palsy, 63
Beta-blockers, 63, 128, 131,
    142–43, 246
Bicycling, 58, 210, 211
Bifocals, 81, 82, 85
Bile, 35, 36, 37, 39
Bile duct, gallstones in, 36, 38,
    40
Biocal, 43
Biofeedback, 50, 51, 52, 129, 130,
    163, 173, 210, 211
Biopsy of prostate gland, 246
Birth control pills. See
    Contraceptives, oral
Birthmarks, 13–14
Blackheads, 282

Blacks
  cancer in, 110
  fibroid tumors in, 247
Bladder, 18, 48, 49, 76, 77, 78, 90,
    95, 107, 112, 247, 252, 256,
    262
Bleeding, 1, 255–56
Blemishes, 279–83
Blepharitis, 63, 66
Blindness from glaucoma, 32
Blood clots, 18, 43
Blood vessels, damaged, 24
Bonding, dental, 285
Bone densitometry, 178, 179,
    180, 182, 183
Bone marrow transplants, 99,
    101, 102, 103, 104, 106,
    107, 108, 109, 110, 111,
    112
Brain injury, posttraumatic, 140
Breathing, 141–42, 158, 161–62,
    171, 174, 223
Bridges, dental, 286–87
Bypass surgery, 5, 7, 8, 9–10, 23,
    59, 60

C
Caffeine, 78, 130–31, 150, 151,
    172, 188
Calcium, 5, 7, 40, 166, 172, 179,
    180, 181, 182
Calcium channel blockers, 79,
    128
Calcium supplements, 42, 43
Camphor-menthol chest rubs,
    230
Cancer, 133, 182
  abdominal cavity, 93
  advances in treatment of,
    89–97
  antibodies for detection of, 89,
    95
  in blacks, 110
  bladder, 18, 90, 95, 112
  bone, 108, 111–12
  brain, 104, 110, 112
  breast, 89, 90–91, 105, 106,
    110, 111, 244–45
  central nervous system, 112
  cervical, 92, 103
  in children, 94, 104, 106, 107

colon, 93, 102, 105, 108
colorectal, 89
early detection of, 91, 113, 122
esophageal, 18, 95, 110
eye, 96
gastrointestinal, 24, 105
genetic research on, 96–97
head and neck, 102, 103, 108, 111
kidney, 105, 108, 110
laser therapy for, 17–18
liver, 93, 109, 110
lung, 18, 95, 102, 110, 112
  test for, 176
nasal, 108
of nerve tissue, 96
obstetric/gynecologic, 111
ovarian, 89, 102, 103, 104, 105, 107, 108, 112, 253
pancreatic, 89, 102, 103, 108, 111–12
prevention of, 91
prostate, 112, 121–23, 246
proton accelerator as treatment for, 89–90
radiation therapy for, 89, 90
skin, 104, 108, 110, 115–20
stomach, 105
testicular, 114
urinary tract, 112
uterine, 92, 105, 255
vaginal, 92
on vocal cords, 16
Cancer treatment centers, 97–114
Carbohydrates, 144–45
Carbon dioxide laser, 12, 15, 16
  for breast cancer surgery, 90–91
Carcinoma, skin, 115, 116, 117
Cataracts, 13, 68, 81, 82
Catheters, 24, 77
CAT scans, 99, 152, 164, 181–82, 183, 187, 253
Cavities, 198, 272
Chemotherapy, 96, 103, 108, 112, 121
  for breast cancer, 244
  intra-arterial, 94, 110
  intraperitoneal, 93–94
Chest pain, 3, 47

Chest rubs, camphor-menthol, 230
Chicken soup, 229–30
Children
  cancer in, 94, 104, 106, 107
  insecurity in, 151
  sun protection for, 118
Chlamydia, 76, 77, 175–76
Cholecystitis, 38
Cholesterol, 3, 18, 19, 26–31, 55, 56, 61, 265. *See also* Plaque, arterial
  in bile, 35, 36, 37
  created by stress, 4
  drugs for, 5–6, 20–21
  and gallstones, 39, 41
  high-density lipoprotein, 21, 28, 29, 30, 31, 79
  increased by antihypertensive medication, 78–80
  intermediary-density lipoprotein, 28
  and intermittent claudication, 58
  levels of, 27, 28, 29, 30, 31
  low-density lipoprotein, 20, 23, 28, 29, 31, 79
  reduced by liposomes, 1
  total, 20, 23, 26–27, 29, 30, 31, 79
  very-low-density lipoprotein, 28
Cirrhosis, 2
Climate and dry-eye syndrome, 62
Clinical trials, 98, 99, 113, 114
Cognitive therapy, 154–55, 156
Colchicine, 2, 44
Colds, 71, 218, 223, 229, 232
Collagen, 67, 68
Community Clinical Oncology Program (CCOP), 100, 101, 113
Condoms, 77, 176
Constipation, 6, 204
Contact lenses, 81, 283
  bifocal, 82
  for color blindness, 87
  for corneal problems, 86–87
  disposable, 86
  for dry eyes, 66–67

Contact lenses (continued)
  eye infection from, 197
  fluorocarbon, 88
  medicated, 86
  ultraviolet-protecting, 83
Continuous positive airway
    pressure (CPAP), 228
Contraceptives, oral, 63, 83, 245,
    249, 256, 257, 271
  causing fibroid growth, 247
  and gallstone formation, 36
  and urinary tract infections, 77
Convulsions in epileptics, 162,
    163, 165
Coronary artery disease, 27, 56,
    60
Cortisone, 236–37, 238, 282
Cosmetic dentists, 287
Cramps
  leg (see Intermittent
    claudication)
  menstrual, 200
Creutzfeldt-Jakob disease, 140
Cryotherapy, 203
Cysts, ovarian, 245

D
Dairy products, 42–43
Dander, 215, 216, 217
Decongestants, 52, 63, 74, 220,
    222, 242, 243
Dementia, 136, 138, 140. See also
    Alzheimer's disease
Dental fillings, 196–97, 283–84
Dental implants, 270–71, 288
Dental sealants, 198
Dentistry, advances in, 283–88
Dentists, cosmetic, 287
Depression, 138, 150, 154, 190
  from digitalis, 124
  after hysterectomy, 251
  winter (see Seasonal affective
    disorder)
Dermabrasion, 14
Dermatitis, 203, 221
Desensitization therapy, 156
Deviated septum, 72, 74, 227
Diabetes, 7, 29, 47, 49, 56, 57, 58,
    61, 139, 143, 262, 263, 271,
    274, 283
Diabetic retinopathy, 12–13

Diaphragm, 77, 176
Diarrhea, 40, 203
Diet, 265
  acne from, 280
  for arterial plaque reduction,
    4, 5, 6
  cholesterol-lowering, 21, 29,
    30, 31
  for epileptics, 171
  for gallstones, 39
  high-fiber, 204
  low-fat, 43
  low-fiber, 91
  vegetarian, 4, 5
Dilantin, 162, 172
Disk, slipped, 206
Diuretics, 52, 63, 246, 271
Down, allergies to, 217
Drops, tear-replacement, 64–65
Drugs. See also individual names of
    drugs
  absorption of, 41, 43, 46, 130
  abuse of, 150
  anti-arthritis, 32
  anticonvulsant, 162, 164, 166,
    172
  antidiarrheal, 203
  antihypertensive, 52, 78–80,
    147, 245–46, 268
  antileukemia, 106
  for arthritis, 46
  as cause of dry-eye syndrome,
    63
  cholesterol-lowering, 5–6,
    20–21, 31, 36, 79
  clot-dissolving, 33
  for dry-eye syndrome, 67–69
  for gallstones, 37, 40–41
  for gout, 44
  for heart, 46
  impotence from, 245–46, 264
  for incontinence, 52–53
  and interaction with alcohol,
    145, 147
  and interaction with food,
    41–47
  for intermittent claudication,
    59
  intra-abdominal delivery of,
    102, 105, 112
  after lithotripsy, 40

nonsteroidal anti-
inflammatory, 235
for pain, 127–28, 130
for panic attacks, 156–57
for Parkinson's disease, 46
for sinusitis, 74
sulfa, 271
sunburn from, 271
Dry-eye syndrome, 61–69
Dual-energy radiography, 182
Dual-photon absorptiometry
(DPA), 181
Dulcolax, 42–43, 45

E
Ear infection, 16
Eczema, 63
Edema, 213, 214
Electroencephalogram, 152, 164,
173
Electrolyte imbalance, 140
Embolism, pulmonary, 43
Endarterectomy, 18, 60, 61
Endometrial ablation, 249, 256
Endometriosis, 251
hysterectomy for, 256–57
laser treatment for, 15
Endorphins, 146
Endoscopy, 1, 24, 38, 75
Epilepsy, 161–74, 262
Epileptic seizures, types of, 165–
66
Ergonomics, 206, 211
Esphesioneuroblastoma (ENB),
108
Estrogen, 36, 53, 69, 180, 182,
183, 245, 247, 249, 252,
254, 256, 257
Estrogen receptors, 245
Eustachian tube blockage, 220
Exercise, 29, 31, 151, 211, 235,
265, 273, 275
for back pain, 206
for epileptics, 174
heel pain from, 234
ice massage before, 204
for incontinence, 48
for intermittent claudication,
57–58, 60
Kegel, 50, 51, 52, 254–55
for loosening phlegm, 232

pelvic muscle, 50, 51
for preventing constipation,
204
for preventing epileptic
seizures, 169
for relaxation, 184–85
strengthening, 208–10
stretching, 208, 235, 237
and symptoms of coronary
artery disease, 56
vision, 85
walking as (see Walking)
Expectorants, 229–31
Eye(s)
allergies affecting, 220, 240
cancer of, 96
diseases of, 81
dry, 61–69
laser surgery for, 12–13
tumors, 90
Eyedrops, 86
Eyelid abnormalities, 63, 67
Eyewear advances, 80–88

F
Fallopian tubes, 34
Familial polyposis, 96
Fascia release, 237–38
Fat, 171
in gallstone diet, 39
polyunsaturated, 118
saturated, 30, 31
Fever, 71, 200, 203, 218
Feverfew, 128–29
Fiber, 171
Fibroids, uterine, 247–49, 251,
252–54, 255
Fibromyomas, 247
Fibronectin, 68–69
Fish oil, 8
Flat feet, 237
Fluoroscope, 6
Folate, 93, 166, 172
Food allergies, 177
Food-drug interactions, 41–47
Foot care with intermittent
claudication, 58
Fractures
hip, 178, 180
pelvic, 262
spinal, 178

Freckles, Retin-A for, 276
Fur, allergies to, 217

G
Gallbladder
  need for, 38–39
  surgery for, 38, 40, 41
Gallstone attacks, 35–36, 38, 39
Gallstones, 34–41
  from aging, 37
  in bile duct, 36, 38, 40
  calcium in, 40
  cholesterol in, 41
  drugs for dissolving, 37
  genetic predisposition to,
    36–37
  lithotripsy for, 40
  in Mexican Americans, 37
  in Native Americans, 36–37
  from obesity, 37
  olive oil for flushing of, 40
  production of, 36
  "silent," 35
  size of, 35
  surgery for, 38, 40, 41
  from weight loss, 37
  in women, 36
Gamma knife, 108, 109
Garden heliotrope. *See* Valerian
Gastritis, 200
Gear, microscopic, 25, 26
Genetics, 22, 36–37, 96–97
Genital warts, 175
Glasses, moisture chamber, 66
Glaucoma, 13, 32–33, 143
Glucose tolerance test, 164
Gonadotropic releasing
    hormone (GnRH), 249,
    254, 257
Gonorrhea, 76, 77
Gout, 2, 44
Grafts for bypass surgery, 9–10,
    60
Grand mal seizure, 162, 163, 165,
    172, 173
Gynecology, lasers in, 15

H
Habit training, for urinary
    incontinence, 52

Hair replacements, 268–69
Hashimoto's disease, 63
Hatha-yoga, 162
Hay fever, 217, 222
Headaches, 200, 204, 216, 221,
    222. *See also* Migraines
Heart, 19–23, 46
Heart attack, 3, 9, 20, 27, 28, 29,
    30, 31, 33, 43, 79, 149, 152,
    155, 225, 248
Heartburn, 200
Heart disease, 22, 56, 59, 118,
    133, 251
Heel pain, 232–38
Help for Incontinent People
    (HIP), 48, 51, 54
Hemangiomas, 14
Hematoporphyrin derivative
    (HpD), 94–95
Hemorrhaging, 44
Hemorrhoids, 203
Hepatitis, 68
Herbal medicine, 78, 143–44
Herpes virus, 76
High blood pressure, 3, 7, 29, 44,
    56, 58, 61, 134, 143, 147,
    225–26, 265, 274
  drugs for, 52, 78–80, 147,
    245–46, 268
High-density lipoprotein (HDL)
    cholesterol, 21, 28, 29, 30,
    31, 79
Hives, 214, 222, 240
Hoarseness, 219
Hodgkin's disease, 103, 109
Hormones, 36, 279–80
Hormone treatment, 256
  for breast cancer, 244, 245
  for endometriosis, 257
  for shrinking fibroids, 254
Hot baths, 146–47, 185
Hot-tip catheter, 9, 18
Humidifiers, 73–74, 230
Humor, for stress reduction,
    148–49
Huntington's disease, 22, 140
Hydrocephalus, 140
Hydrolyzed vegetable protein,
    132, 133
Hyperthermia, 102, 106, 110
Hyperthyroidism, 140

Hyperventilation, 154, 155, 156, 158
Hypochondria, 152
Hypoglycemia, 164
Hypothyroidism, 140
Hypoventilation, 155
Hysterectomy, 16, 53, 92, 125, 248, 249–59
Hysteroscope, 253

I

Ibuprofen, 127, 200, 201
Ice massage, 235, 236, 237
Ice packs, 203–4
Ileostomy, 107
Implants
    dental, 270–71, 288
    penile, 263–64
Impotence, 245–46, 260–65
Incontinence, urinary, 47–54, 122
    behavioral therapy for, 50–52
    help for, 53–54
    hysterectomy for, 259
    medical treatment for, 52–53
    patterns of, 49–50
    surgery for, 47, 48, 53
    from vitamin B_{12} deficiency, 192
Indigestion, 200
Infections, 255
    antibiotics for, 42
    from blocked bile duct, 36
    eye, 67, 86, 87, 197
    with intermittent claudication, 57, 58, 59
    kidney, 76
    in laser surgery, 12
    respiratory (see Colds)
    sinus (see Sinusitis)
    urinary tract, 49, 75–78
    from vitamin B_{12} deficiency, 190
Infertility, 15, 175, 247, 248
Injuries, spinal cord, 49, 50, 262, 263
Insect bites, 203, 204, 214
Insomnia, 150
Insulin, 139, 144
Intercourse, 76, 77, 78, 175

Intermediary-density lipoprotein (IDL), 28
Intermittent claudication, 54–61
Iridotomy, 13
Iron supplements, 46
Irritable bowel syndrome, 39
Isoniazid, 44, 45, 46
Itching, 221, 240
IUD, 255

K

Kegel exercises, 50, 51, 52, 254–55
Keratoconjunctivitis sicca. See Dry-eye syndrome
Keratoses, Retin-A for, 276
Kidneys, 48, 76, 96, 140, 252, 262
Kidney stones, 17, 44

L

Laminates, dental, 284–86
Laparoscopy, 15, 253, 257
Laser, 11–18
    for ablation of endometrium, 249, 256
    in angioplasty, 8
    argon, 11–12, 13, 14, 15
    for cancer treatment, 17–18
    carbon dioxide, 12, 15, 16
        for breast cancer surgery, 90–91
    drug treatment combined with, 94–95
    in gynecology, 15
    for intermittent claudication, 60
    after lithotripsy for kidney stones, 17
    for lung cancer surgery, 112
    neodymium-YAG, 12, 13, 16
    for punctal occlusion, 67
    for tattoo removal, 14–15
    tunable-dye, 12, 14
Laser endarterectomy, 18
Laser surgery
    for endometriosis, 257
    for eyes, 12–13
    for glaucoma, 33
    for skin, 13–14
Laser trabeculoplasty, 13
Lateral tarsorrhaphy, 67

Laxatives, 42–43, 204
Leiomyomas, 247
Leukemia, 103, 106, 107, 109,
    111, 112
  childhood, 101
  chronic myelocytic, 96
  hairy cell, 110, 112
Levodopa, 45, 46
Lifestyle, cholesterol-lowering,
    4–6
Lipoproteins, 19, 20, 28
Liposomes, 1, 2
Liposuction, 272–75
Lithotripsy, 17, 40
Liver
  damaged, 40
  disorders of, 262
  failure of, 140
Low-density lipoprotein (LDL)
    cholesterol, 20, 21, 23, 28,
    29, 31, 79
Lozenges, 230
Lupus, 64
Lymphoma, 103, 106, 107, 109,
    111, 112

M
Macrophages, 19, 20
Magnetic resonance imaging
    (MRI), 21, 99, 187
Mastoid disease, 16
Medical tests, anxiety before,
    183–89
Medications. See Drugs
Meditation, 162, 173, 185
Melanoma, 104, 105, 108, 110,
    111, 112, 115, 116, 117,
    120, 160
Memory loss, 189, 190
Meningitis, 140
Menopause, 151, 178, 180, 182,
    247, 252, 254, 255, 256
  premature, 179, 182
Menstruation, 248, 249, 255–56
Meprobamates, 147, 148
Mexican Americans, gallstones
    in, 37
Microdynamics, 24, 25
Microgear, 25, 26
Micromachines, 24
Middle ear infection, 16

Migraines, 126–33, 221
Milk, 42, 43, 130
Minipress, 79, 80
Minoxidil, 265–68
Miscarriage, 248
Moisture-chamber glasses, 66
Mold, 73, 243
Moles, 116, 120
Monoamine oxidase inhibitors
    (MAOIs), 157
Monosodium glutamate (MSG),
    and migraines, 132–33
Mucus, 219, 223. See also Phlegm
Multiple sclerosis, 49, 140
Music for migraines, 129–30
Mycosis fungoides, 102
Myelin, 190
Myeloma, multiple, 111
Myofascial syndrome, 206
Myomectomy, 248, 253–54
Myopia, 87

N
Nasal conditions, 16, 177, 214,
    221, 227, 240
Nasal sprays, 220
National Cancer Institute
    treatment centers, 97–114
National Cholesterol Education
    Program (NCEP), 29
Native Americans, gallstones in,
    36–37
Nearsightedness, 87
Negative-ion generators, 73
Neodymium-YAG laser, 12, 13,
    16
Neuroblastoma, 96
Neuroma, acoustic, 16–17
Neurosyphilis, 140
Nicotine, 131, 172
Nosebleeds, 16

O
Obesity, 22, 29, 37, 58, 273
Ointment
  antibiotic, 201–2
  boric acid, 221
  tear-replacement, 65–66
Olive oil, 40
Omnipen, 42, 45
Oncogenes, 96

Oophorectomy, 179, 250, 257
Ophthalmologists, 87
Opticians, 87
Optometrists, 87
Organ transplants, 69
Orthokeratology, 87–88
Orthotic shoe inserts, 234, 237
Osteoarthritis, drug for, 32
Osteogenic sarcoma, 94
Osteoporosis screening, 178–83
Ostomies, 107
Otitis media, 220
Ovarian cysts, 245
Ovaries, 252–53, 256, 257
Oxalates, 43
Ozone depletion, 117

P
Pacemakers, 2–3
Pain
    back, 205–12
    chest, 3, 47
    from gallstones, 35–36, 38, 39
    from gout, 44
    heel, 232–38
    ice for relief of, 204
    from intermittent
        claudication, 55, 57
    migraine (*see* Migraines)
    from nasal congestion, 221
    pelvic, 248, 258–59
    reduced, after breast surgery,
        91
    sinus, 214
    from sinusitis, 71
Painkillers, 127–28, 130
Palladium capsules, 121–23
Pancreatitis, 38, 39
Panic attacks, 149–58
Pan-retinal photocoagulation, 12
Papilloma virus, 15
Pap smear, 175
Parkinson's disease, 46, 49, 262
Pelvic inflammatory disease, 175
Pelvic muscle exercises. *See*
    Kegel exercises
Pelvic pain, 248, 258–59
Pelvic tilt, 209
Penicillin, 42, 45
Penile implants, 263–64
Penile injections, 263

Peripheral vascular disease, 56
Pessary, 255
Pesticides, 172
Petit mal seizure, 163, 165, 167
Petrolatum, 199, 220, 221
Pets, allergies to, 215
Peyronie's disease, 262
Phlegm, 228–32. *See also* Mucus
Phobias, 152–53, 155, 158
Phototherapy, for seasonal
    affective disorder, 160–61
Physical therapy, 237
Physician Data Query (PDQ),
    98, 101
Phytic acid, 43
Pick's disease, 140
Pillows, allergies to, 216
Plantar fasciitis, 233–38
Plaque
    arterial, 3–10, 19, 20, 55, 61,
        262 (*see also* Cholesterol)
        balloon angioplasty for,
            6–8, 9, 10
        diet for, 4, 5, 6
        drugs for, 5–6
        laser for, 9, 18
        lifestyle changes for, 4–6
        prevention of, 3
        reduced by liposomes, 1–2
        surgery for, 9–10
    dental, 272
Plaquenil, 67–68
Pneumonia, 232
Pollen, 73, 213, 215, 221, 222, 243
Pollution, 72–73
Polyps, 16
Polyunsaturated fat, 118
Port-wine stains, 13–14
Postnasal drip, 71, 219
Precancerous lesions, 13, 15
Pregnancy, 257
    ectopic, 175
    in epileptics, 168
    fibroids during, 247
    and gallstone formation, 36
    Kegel exercises after, 50
    prevented by fibroids, 248
    urinary tract infections
        during, 76
Presbyopia, 81–82
Priapism, 262

Procainamide, 45, 46
Progesterone, 249, 256
Progressive addition lenses, 81
Progressive muscle relaxation, 129, 142, 169, 170, 185
Pronation, 233
Prostate gland, 49, 50, 80, 262
 blockages of, 34
 cancer of, 112, 121–23, 246
 surgery for, 53
 treatment of, 34, 246, 254
Prostheses, 24, 108
Proton accelerator, 89–90
Psoriasis, 63
Psychotherapy
 for epileptics, 173
 for impotence, 261, 264
 for panic attacks, 155–56
 for pelvic pain sufferers, 259
Punctal occlusion, 67
Purines, 44

R
Radial keratotomy, 88
Radiation therapy, 89, 90, 92, 94, 102, 103, 105, 106, 108, 109, 110, 111, 121
Relaxation, 185, 188
Relaxation response, 162–63, 171
Resin dental fillings, 196–97, 284
Restenosis, 7, 8
Retin-A, 276–79, 282
Retina, 12–13, 82
Retinoblastoma, 96
Retinoic acid, 278, 279
Retinopathy, diabetic, 12–13
Reye's syndrome, 200
Rheumatoid arthritis, 32, 64, 134
Rhinitis, 214, 217, 218
Rhinorrhea, 240
Riley-Day syndrome, 63
Rogaine Topical Solution. *See* Minoxidil
Running, 235

S
Salt, 202–3
Saturated fat, 30, 31
Scalp reduction, 268
Seasonal affective disorder, 159–61

Seizures, epileptic, 165–66
Seldane, 240–41
Septum, deviated, 72, 74, 218–19, 227
Serotonin, 126, 127, 128, 144
Sex. *See* Intercourse
Sex therapy, 261, 264
Sexual dysfunction
 after hysterectomy, 251
 in men (*see* Impotence)
Sexually transmitted diseases, 76, 77, 175
Shoes, 235
Silicone, 53, 67
Simon Foundation for Continence, 54
Single photon absorptiometry (SPA), 181
Sinuses, blocked, 222
Sinusitis, 70–75
Sit-ups, 209
Six-three-six method, to slow breathing, 141–42
Sjogren's syndrome, 63–64, 67, 68
Skin tests, 222
Sleep apnea. *See* Apnea, sleep
Sleeping pills, 52, 63, 227
 natural, 144
Smoking, 3, 4, 22, 29, 31, 55, 57, 60, 61, 73, 91, 131, 182, 214, 262, 265, 274
Snoring, 224–28
Spermicide, 77
Sphincter muscles, 48, 49, 52, 53
Sphincterotomy, 38
Spicy foods, 230–31
Spider veins, 14
Spina bifida, 53
Spinal cord injuries, 49, 50, 262, 263
Stapedectomy, 17
Static electricity, 25–26
Stress, 4, 140–49, 262, 280. *See also* Anxiety; Panic attacks
Stretching, 208, 235, 237
Stroke, 3, 9, 20, 43, 50, 133, 134, 140, 152, 155, 182, 225
Stroke dementia, 125–26
Subliminal messages during surgery, 124–25

Sugarless gum, 271–72
Sumycin, 42, 45
Sun, acne from, 280
Sunburn, 160, 203, 271, 278
Sun exposure, 91, 117–20
Sunglasses, 83–84
Sunscreen, 119, 271, 277
Supplements
    calcium, 42, 43
    for epileptics, 171, 172
    iron, 46
    thyroid, 43
Surgery
    bladder, 262
    brain, 108, 109, 110
    breast, 90–91, 111, 244
    bypass, 5, 7, 8, 9–10, 23, 59, 60
    cataract, 68, 82
    catheters for, 24
    coronary bypass, 23
    for deviated septum, 74–75,
        218–19, 227
    for dry-eye syndrome, 67
    endoscopic, 24
    eye, 63
    fascia release, 237–38
    foot, 234
    gallbladder, 34, 38, 40
    for impotence, 263
    for incontinence, 47, 48, 53
    for intermittent claudication,
        59–61
    kidney, 17
    laser, 11–18, 33, 90–91, 257
    prostate, 53, 80, 121, 262
    rectal, 262
    subliminal messages during,
        124–25
    suspension, 53
    voice-saving, 108
Swimming, 58, 235
Sympathectomy, 60–61

T
Tanning booths, 120
Taping, foot, 235–36
Tattoo removal, 14–15
Tear replacements, 64–66
Tempeh, 194
Tension. See Anxiety; Panic
    attacks; Stress

Testing, medical
    anxiety before, 183–89
    noninvasive, 21
Testosterone, 261, 262
Tetracycline, 42, 45, 83, 271
Tetrahydroaminoacridine, 139
Tetrex, 42, 45
Therapy. See individual types of
    therapy
Thrombophlebitis, 43
Thyroid supplements, 43
Tobacco, 72–73, 214, 265
Tongue-retaining device, 227
Tonsillectomy, 12, 275
Toothaches, 200
Total cholesterol, 26–27, 29, 30,
    31
Tranquilizers, 63, 141, 143–48,
    227
Tretinoin. See Retin-A
Trifocals, 81, 85
Trigger-point injection, 259
Triglycerides, 28, 30
Tuberculosis, 44, 90
Tumor necrosis factor, 96
Tumors
    bone, 94, 110
    brain, 16, 90, 102, 103, 104,
        106, 140, 152, 154
    drug-laser removal of,
        94–95
    eye, 90
    fibroid, 247–49, 251, 252–54,
        255
    kidney, 96
    malignant, 89
    pancreatic, 24
    spinal, 90
    in windpipe, 16
Tunable-dye lasers, 12, 14
Tyramine, 44

U
Ulcers, 1, 39, 200
Ultrasound, 24
    B-mode, for monitoring
        atherosclerosis, 21
    for fibroid assessment, 248
    for glaucoma, 32–33
    for ovary assessment, 253
    for prostate gland, 122, 246

Ultraviolet light, 82–83, 116, 117, 118, 119, 120, 160
University of Miami's Comprehensive Pain and Rehabilitation Center, 205, 206
Ureters, 48, 49
Urethra, 48, 49, 75, 76
Uric acid, 44
Urinalysis, 76, 77
Urinary incontinence. *See* Incontinence, urinary
Urinary system, 48–49, 51
Urinary tract infections, 49, 75–78
Ursodiol, 37, 40–41
Uterine fibroids, 247–49, 251, 252–54, 255
Uterine prolapse, 251, 254–55
Uvulopalatopharyngoplasty (UPPP), 228

V
Vagina, 75, 78, 92
Vaginitis, 202–3
Valerian, 143–44
Valium, 147, 148, 157
Vaporizers, 230
Vascular disease, 18, 20, 21
Very-low-density lipoprotein (VLDL), 28

Video display terminals, 62–63, 85–86
Videolaseroscopy, 257
Vision therapy, 85
Visualization, 129, 130, 156, 185, 187–88
Vitamin B complex, 172
Vitamin B_6, 172
Vitamin B_{12}, 172, 189–95
Vitamin D, 166, 172
Vitamin E, 59
Vitamin K, 43–44
Vocal cords, polyps on, 16

W
Walking, 57–58, 60, 145–46, 158, 169, 184–85, 211, 234, 235
Warts, 13, 15, 175
Water, 74, 76, 204, 219, 229
Weight loss, 37, 58, 226–27
Wilms' tumor, 96
Windpipe, tumors obstructing, 16
Women
    gallstones in, 36
    panic attacks in, 151
    seasonal affective disorder in, 159
Wool, allergies to, 216
Wrinkles, Retin-A for, 276, 278